Lange Instant Access: Orthopedics and Sports Medicine

MVFOL

D0401385

Lange Instant Access: Orthopedics and Sports Medicine

Anil M. Patel, MD
Adjunct Assistant Professor
Family Medicine Physician
Touro University Nevada College of Osteopathic Medicine
Henderson, Nevada
Residency completion: University of Pittsburgh Medical Center (UPMC)
Pittsburgh, Pennsylvania

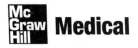 **Medical**

New York   Chicago   San Francisco   Lisbon   London
Madrid   Mexico City   New Delhi   San Juan   Seoul
Singapore   Sydney   Toronto

The McGraw·Hill Companies

Lange Instant Access:
Orthopedics and Sports Medicine

1 2 3 4 5 6 7 8 9 0   DOC/DOC   0 9 8 7

ISBN 978-0-07-149009-2
MHID 0-07-149009-4

This book was set in Palatino by International Typesetting and Composition.
The editor was Jim Shanahan.
The production supervisor was Sherri Souffrance.
Project management was provided by International Typesetting
    and Composition.
RR Donnelley was printer and binder.
This book is printed on acid-free paper.

Cataloging-in-Publication data for this title is on file with the
Library of Congress.

Contents

Author

Anil M. Patel, MD
Adjunct Assistant Professor
Family Medicine Physician
Touro University Nevada College of Osteopathic Medicine
Henderson, Nevada
Residency completion: University of Pittsburgh Medical Center
Pittsburgh, Pennsylvania (UPMC)

Editors and Contributors

Evelyn Omana, MD
University of Pittsburgh Medical Center (UPMC)
Family Medicine Residency Program, PGY III
Pittsburgh, Pennsylvania

Dipti Patel, DO
Family Medicine Physician
Urgent Care/Primary Care Clinic
Residency completion: University of Pittsburgh Medical Center
(UPMC)

Phoebe Tobiano, MD
Family Medicine Physician
Private Practice
Residency completion: University of Pittsburgh Medical Center
(UPMC)

Preface

This book presents essential facts and data that inherently are a part of the patient care encounters faced by new clinicians. It was written to be used independently, but can be used as a companion to a standard handbook of sports medicine and orthopedic medicine. This book's main focus is on step by step guidance to the clinical method of diagnosis and treatment. *Lange Instant Access: Orthopedics and Sports Medicine* presents the high-yield facts and data that underlie patient presentations and disease and clinical interventions.

Lange Instant Access: Orthopedics and Sports Medicine was written for third and fourth year medical students and interns. It includes information essential for today's learning. It covers multiple topics in orthopedics and sports medicine. The content of each chapter was based on the most commonly asked questions among medical students and interns. All the materials were acquired from respected references in medical literature.

This book, a product of one and a half years of hard work, was reviewed by physicians respected in their fields.

This book will be helpful to all in their journey to becoming a great physician.

Acknowledgments

I would like to dedicate *Lange Instant Access: Orthopedics and Sports Medicine* to my grandmother who influenced me in becoming a physician. I would like to thank all the editors and contributors for their time and hard work devoted to this book; without their effort this manual would not be possible. I also would like to thank James Shanahan, Patti Bearley, Laura Libretti, and Aparna Shukla and her team for working very closely with me in making *Lange Instant Access: Orthopedics and Sports Medicine* a reality.

Anil M. Patel, MD

1
Guide

TABLE 1–1: Common Abbreviations	
AC	Acromioclavicular
A-P	Antero-posterior
Blood C&S	Blood culture and sensitivity
CBC	Complete blood count
CPK	Creatinine phosphokinase
CRP	C-reactive protein
CT	Computer tomography
CTS	Carpal tunnel syndrome
EMG	Electromyogram
ESR	Erythrocyte sedementation rate
MRI	Magnetic resonance imaging
NCS	Nerve conduction study
NSAIDS	Nonsteroidal anti-inflammatory drugs
ORIF	Open reduction internal fixation
PSA	Prostatic specific antigen
TENS	Transcutaneous electrical nerve stimulation

TABLE 1–2: Motor: Muscle Strength Grading
0/5—No muscle contraction noted
1/5—Muscle contraction, visible or palpable but no movement
2/5—Movement with gravity eliminated
3/5—Movement with gravity
4/5—Movement against gravity with some resistance
5/5—Movement against gravity with resistance (normal strength)

TABLE 1–3: Major Nerves and Their Actions		
Upper Extremities		
Nerve	**Sensation**	**Motor**
Axillary	Lateral shoulder	Shoulder abduction
Musculocutaneous	Lateral forearm	Elbow flexion
Median	Lateral palm	Thumb opposition
Radial	Dorsolateral hand	Finger extension
Ulnar	Medial hand	Finger abduction/ adduction
Lower Extremities		
Obturator	Medial thigh	Thigh adduction
Femoral	Anterior thigh	Knee extension
Sciatic	Posterolateral calf	Knee flexion
Peroneal	Dorsal foot	Toe extension
Tibial	Plantar foot	Toe flexion

TABLE 1–4: Deep Tendon Reflexes
0—Absent reflex
1+—Hypoactive
2+—Normal
3+—Brisker than average
4+—Hyperactive

TABLE 1–5: Neurological Reflexes	
Muscle reflex	**Spinal roots**
Biceps stretch	C5–C6
Brachioradialis	C5–C6
Finger flexor (=Hoffman's sign)	C6–C7
Triceps stretch	C7–C8
Hamstrings (medial and lateral)	L5–S2
Patellar (knee jerk)	L2–L4
Achilles (ankle jerk)	S1–S2

TABLE 1–6: Laceration Guideline				
Immunization status	**Clean, minor wound**		**All other wound**	
	Td	**TIG**	**Td**	**TIG**
≥3 doses received in immunization series	Give only if last booster >10 yrs	No	If last booster >5 yrs	No*
<3 doses received or uncertain of immunization	Yes	No	Yes	Yes

*TIG is not given unless patient has humoral immune deficiency (e.g., HIV, agammaglobulinemia).

Tetanus toxoid dosage 0.5-mg IM × 1 dose.

Td and TIG should be given on two separate sites.

TIG = tetanus immunoglobulin.   Td = tetanus toxoid.

Source: *MMWR Morb Mortal Wkly Rep.* 1991, 40(RR-10): 1.

TABLE 1–7: Salter–Harris Fractures	
Types	**Area involved**
I	Epiphyseal separation only
II	Fracture in metaphysis with displacement of epiphysis
III	Fracture thru epiphysis and growth plate
IV	Fracture through epiphysis, growth plate, and into metaphysis
V	Injury to epiphysis and plate

TABLE 1–8: Synovial Fluid Analysis

Description	Normal	Septic	Inflammatory	Noninflammatory	Hemorrhagic
Color	Clear	Yellow-green	Yellow	Yellow	Red
Viscosity	High	Variable	Low	High	Variable
WBC/mm^3	<200 K	>75 K	25–50 K	<10 K	<10 K
PMNs (%)	<25	>75	>50	<25	50–75
Glucose (mg/dL)	Same as serum	<25	>25	Same as serum	Same as serum
Protein (g/dL)	1–2	3–5	3–5	1–3	4–6
LDH (compared to serum)	Very low	Variable	High	Very low	Same as serum

PMN – Polymorphonuclear neutrophils
LDH – Lactate dehydrogenase

FIGURES 1–1 to 1–10: Range of Motion

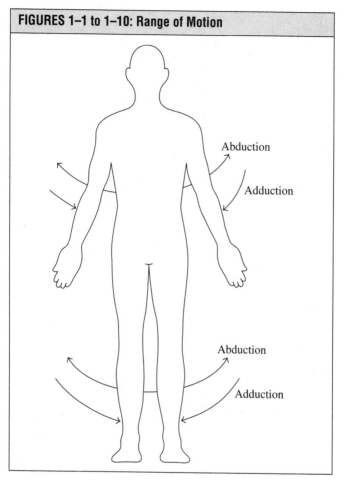

Abduction

Adduction

Abduction

Adduction

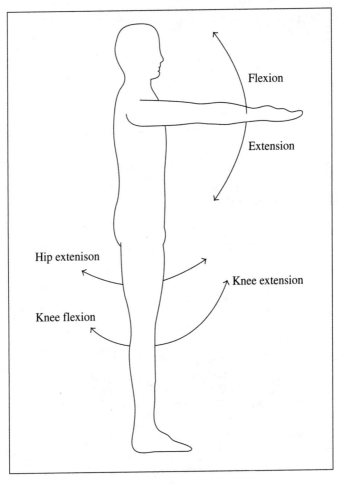

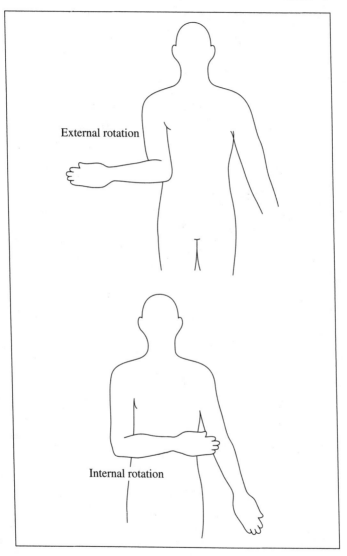

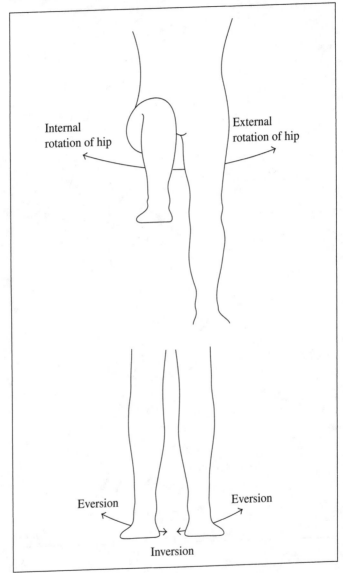

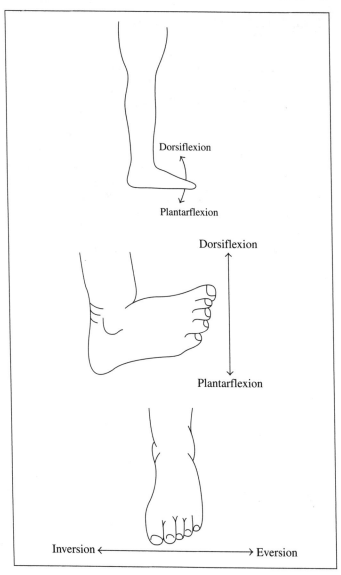

FIGURE 1–2: Sensory: Dermatomal Map

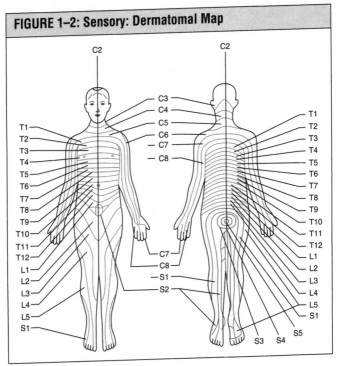

FIGURE 2–1: Anatomy

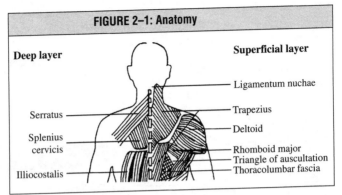

Deep layer

Serratus

Splenius cervicis

Illiocostalis

Superficial layer

Ligamentum nuchae

Trapezius

Deltoid

Rhomboid major
Triangle of auscultation
Thoracolumbar fascia

TABLE 2–1: Assessment of Injury

A. Detailed history

B. Inspection: Swelling, erythema, discoloration, deformity, laceration

C. Palpation: Bones and soft tissue—tenderness, deformity, effusion

D. Range of motion: Passive and active

Neck Muscle Actions	
Flexion (chin to chest)	**Extension (looking up the sky)**
(1) Longus coli	(1) Spinous capitis
(2) Longus capitus	(2) Semispinalis capitis
(3) Infrahyoid	(3) Suboccipital (rectus capitis posterior major and minor, obliquus capitis superior and inferior)
	(4) Trapezius
Lateral rotation	**Lateral flexion**
(1) Splenius capitis	(1) Scalenes

(continued)

TABLE 2–1: Assessment of Injury (Continued)

(2) Sternocleidomastoid	
(3) Levator scapula	
(4) Suboccipital (rectus capitis posterior major and minor, obliquus capitis superior and inferior)	

Cervical Level and Its Corresponding Function

Nerve root	Functional finding	Corresponding muscles
C4	Shoulder elevation	Levator scapular and trapezius
C5	Shoulder abduction and external rotation	Rhomboid, deltoid, biceps, and infraspinatus
C6	Flexion at elbow, shoulder external rotation	Infraspinatus, biceps, brachioradialis,
	Bicep/brachioradialis reflex	Pronator teres, and triceps
C7	Elbow extensors, forearm pronators	Triceps, pronator teres, flexor carpi radialis
	Triceps reflex	
C8	Finger abductors and grip strength	

(continued)

TABLE 2–1: Assessment of Injury (Continued)
• **Motor** (see Chapter 1)
• **Sensory** (see Chapter 1)
• **Deep tendon reflex** (see Chapter 1)
• **Vascular** (check distal pulses)
• **Red flags**
• Bowel or bladder dysfunction or weakness
• Neurological dysfunction
• History of malignancy
• Cauda equina syndrome
• Age >50 yrs
• Fever
• Unintentional weight loss

TABLE 2–2: Diagnostic Approaches
Imaging studies
• **AP and lateral**
• **Swimmer's view** (to visualize C7)
• **CT:** Can detect degenerative changes, disc herniation, central and foramen stenosis, osteoarthritis, tumor, and fractures.
• **MRI:** More sensitive for soft tissue and malignancy. Also useful in herniation, central, and foramen stenosis. Gadolinium contrast offers better diagnosis of infection, malignancy, or post surgical fibrosis. (Avoid gadolinium if glomerular filtration rate <15–30 mL/min).
Lab studies
• CBC with diff
• Blood C&S
• ESR
• CRP
Other studies
• **EMG:** Useful when peripheral nerve entrapment is suspected.
• **NCS:** Useful test to identify cervical radiculopathy.
• **Myelogram:** Useful in identifying defect with spinal cord, spinal canal, spinal nerve root and blood vessel, and arachnoid membrane.

TABLE 2–3: Common Conditions and Management

A. Cervical Discogenic Pain: Is a radiological diagnosis.
Clinical: May or may not be symptomatic.
Neck pain with or without inflammation; exacerbated by placing neck in a prolonged position such as driving, studying, using computer, etc.
May have decreased range of motion; no neurological deficit.
Management: Oral anti-inflammatory medication, physical therapy, surgery.
B. Cervical Facet Syndrome
Clinical: Some history of abrupt flexion-extension type of injury or repeatedly positioning neck in extension.
Midline neck pain, radiating to shoulders.
Management: A fluoroscopic guided intra-articular injection of local anesthetic can be diagnostic as well as therapeutic.
C. Cervical Myofascial Pain: A localized pain with trigger points associated with stiff bands, and pressure sensitivity.
Clinical: May be a nonspecific manifestation of a pathological condition.
May be associated with depression, insomnia, and fibromyalgia.
Management: Anti-inflammatory medication, physical therapy/exercise, trigger point (local anesthetic) injection.
D. Cervical Radiculopathy
Etiology: Degenerative changes, foramen stenosis, herniated disc, zoster, diabetic neuropathy, Lyme disease
Clinical: Tingling and numbness over arm or fingers in a dermatomal pattern, usually unilateral.
Central disc herniation can cause myelopathy (bilateral weakness, spasticity, increased tendon reflexes, Babinski responses); may have urinary urgency, incontinence, or urinary retention.

(continued)

TABLE 2–3: Common Conditions and Management (Continued)

Management: Ice, anti-inflammatory medication, physical therapy, cervical epidural steroid.

E. Cervical Spine Fracture

Etiology: Are common with fall from height, diving accident, or motor vehicle accident.

Clinical: Presents as intense neck pain with muscle spasm and point tenderness. A step-off (a radiologic finding) between spinous processes represents an injury to posterior ligamentous complex, which is considered unstable.

Management: Immobilization, steroids IV (Methylprednisolone 30 mg/kg IV q30min; followed by continuous IV drip 5.4 mg/kg q1h for 24hours).

F. Cervical Spondylosis: A degenerative changes of the spine noted on radiograph which includes changes in the intervertebral discs, with formation of the osteophytes along the vertebral bodies, changes in the facet joints and laminal arches.

Clinical: Neck pain, stiffness, radicular signs.

Management: Immobilization, pharmacologic treatments, physical therapy (traction, manipulation, exercises).

G. Cervical Spondylotic Myelopathy: Degenerative changes narrowing the spinal canal leading to spinal cord injury and dysfunction.

Etiology: Due to an extradural mass such as herniated nucleus pulposus, posterior longitudinal ligament ossification, spondylolisthesis, subaxial cervical instability due to rheumatoid arthritis, degenerative C1 to C2, congenital narrowing, or endplate hyperostosis.

Clinical: Neck stiffness, crepitus with neck movement, brachiaglia, dull aching pain in arm, numbness/tingling in hands

Management: Immobilization, physical therapy (traction, exercises), surgery

(continued)

TABLE 2–3: Common Conditions and Management (Continued)

H. Cervical Strain
Etiology: Due to physical stress, poor posture, improper neck position, and poor sleeping habits. Injury to paraspinal muscles and ligaments associated with muscle spasms of the cervical and upper back.
Clinical: Presents as a muscle pain, stiffness, and tightness over upper back, neck, or shoulder.
The pain can last up to 6 weeks.
Management: Reassurance, muscle relaxant, anti-inflammatory medication, cervical collar.
Doxepin or Amitriptyline may be helpful with sleeping difficulty.
I. Diffuse Idiopathic Skeletal Hyperostosis: Is a inappropriate bone dumping in the ligaments and tendons
Diagnostic criteria:
(1) Ossification and calcification found along the anterolateral aspects of ≥4 contiguous vertebrae
(2) Relative conservation of intervertebral disc height without widespread changes of primary degenerative disc disease
(3) Absence of apophyseal joint ankylosing or sacroiliac joint erosion, sclerosis, or intra-articular ankylosis
Clinical: Is associated with pain, stiffness, and loss of mobility.
Management: Anti-inflammatory medication, physical therapy
J. Thoracic Outlet Syndrome
Clinical: Neck and shoulder pain radiating to arms.
Triad: Weakness, numbness, and sensation of swelling of the arms

(continued)

TABLE 2–3: Common Conditions and Management (Continued)
Roos sign: Positive.
Individual elevates, abducts, and externally rotates both arms. Individual holds the position while repeatedly opening and closing the hands for about 3 minutes. Reproduction of the symptoms is a positive test.
Management: Physical therapy, surgery
K. Whiplash Injury
Etiology: Due to an abrupt flexion-extension of the neck, most commonly after trauma
Clinical: Spasm, pain, loss of range of motion, headache; may have injury to soft tissues, intervertebral disc, spinal nerve, posterior longitudinal ligament, or facet joint
Management: Rest, anti-inflammatory medication, muscle relaxants for 2–4 weeks

TABLE 2–4: Special Tests
Spurling test
• **Indication:** To assess cervical root disorder
• **Technique:** Spine extended with head rotated to affected shoulder while axially loaded
• **Interpretation:** Reproduction of radicular pain = cervical nerve root compression

FIGURE 2–2: Spurling Test

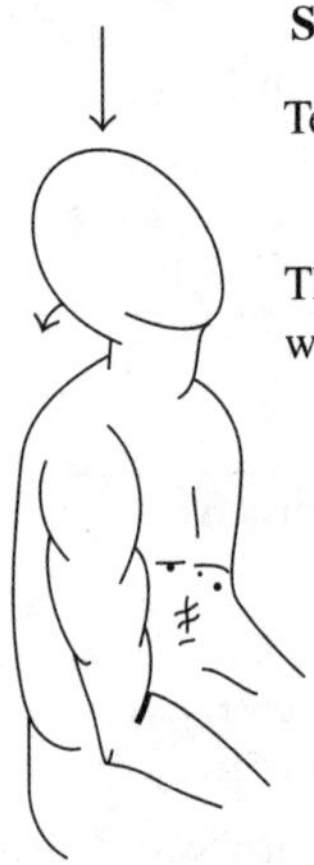

Spurling test

Testing for cervical root disorders

The neck is extended and rotated laterally while and axial load is placed on spine

3
Shoulder

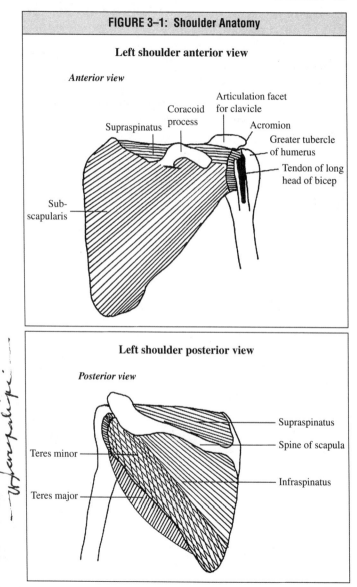

FIGURE 3–1: Shoulder Anatomy

Left shoulder anterior view

Anterior view

Supraspinatus

Coracoid process

Articulation facet for clavicle

Acromion

Greater tubercle of humerus

Tendon of long head of bicep

Sub-scapularis

Left shoulder posterior view

Posterior view

Teres minor

Teres major

Supraspinatus

Spine of scapula

Infraspinatus

(continued)

FIGURE 3–1: Shoulder Anatomy

Left shoulder anterior view

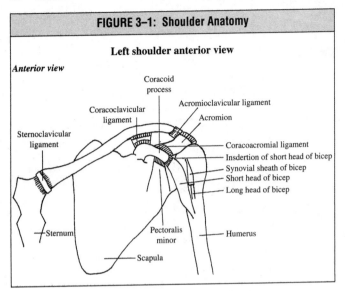

Anterior view

Coracoid process

Coracoclavicular ligament

Acromioclavicular ligament

Acromion

Coracoacromial ligament

Insdertion of short head of bicep

Synovial sheath of bicep

Short head of bicep

Long head of bicep

Sternoclavicular ligament

Sternum

Pectoralis minor

Humerus

Scapula

Brachial plexus

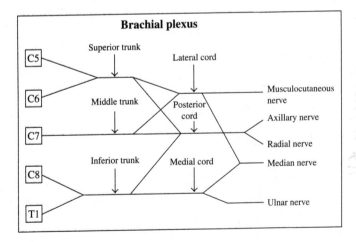

Superior trunk

Lateral cord

C5

C6

Middle trunk

Posterior cord

Musculocutaneous nerve

C7

Axillary nerve

Radial nerve

Inferior trunk

Medial cord

Median nerve

C8

T1

Ulnar nerve

TABLE 3–1: Assessment of Injury

A. Detailed history

B. Inspection: Swelling, erythema, discoloration, deformity, laceration

C. Palpation: Bones and soft tissue—tenderness, deformity, effusion, soft tissue

D. Range of motion: Passive and active

Normal Shoulder Range of Motion

Action	Degrees
Flexion	135
Extension	45
Abduction	180
Adduction	45
Internal rotation	70
External rotation	45

Shoulder Range of Motion and Muscle Actions

Flexion	Extension
Primary	Primary
(1) Deltoid	(1) Latissimus dorsi
(2) Coracobrachialis	(2) Teres major
	(3) Deltoid
Secondary	**Secondary**
(1) Pectoralis major	(1) Teres minor
(2) Bicep	(2) Triceps
(3) Deltoid	
Internal rotation	**External rotation**
Latissimus dorsi	Deltoid
Pectoralis major	Infraspinatus

(continued)

TABLE 3–1: Assessment of Injury (Continued)	
Teres major	Teres minor
Deltoid	
Subscapularis	
Adduction	**Abduction**
Latissimus dorsi	Deltoid
Pectoralis major	Supraspinatus
Teres major	Pectoralis major
Coracobrachialis	
Triceps brachii	
Transverse flexion	**Transverse flexion**
Pectoralis major	Deltoid
Deltoid	Latissimus dorsi
Coracobrachialis	Infraspinatus
Bicep brachii	Teres minor
Tranverse adduction	**Transverse abduction**
Pectoralis major	Deltoid
Coracobrachialis	Infraspinatus
	Teres minor
• Motor (see Chapter 1)	
• Sensory (see Chapter 1)	
• Deep tendon reflexes (see Chapter 1)	
• Vascular (check distal pulses)	

TABLE 3–2: Localization of the Pain
Anterolateral Shoulder Pain
• Impingement syndrome (especially when aggravated by reaching overhead)
• Rotator cuff tendinitis
• Rotator cuff tear
• Adhesive Capsulitis ("frozen shoulder"); stiffness and loss of external rotation and abduction
• AC joint separation
• Osteoarthritis
• Glenohumeral Joint Injury
• Bicep Muscle Injury
Posterior Shoulder Pain
• Rotator Cuff Tendinitis
• Cervical Strain
• Radiculopathy
• Extraglenohumeral Etiology
• Extrinsic Shoulder Etiology

TABLE 3–3: Diagnostic Approaches

Clinical

- Assess traumatic vs. nontraumatic
- Intrinsic shoulder vs. extrinsic (cervical root, abdominal etc.)
- If intrinsic shoulder, assess glenohumeral vs. extraglenohumeral

Glenohumeral

- Rotator cuff injury (tear, tendinitis)
- Impingement
- Adhesive capsulitis
- Glenohumeral osteoarthritis
- Multidirectional shoulder instability

Imaging Studies

- Shoulder radiograph: AP and axillary view, transscapular if unable to perform axillary view
- MRI: Especially if impingement and rotator cuff injury suspected
- Ultrasonography: Diagnosing rotator cuff injury, labral tear, bicep tendon tear, or dislocation; this modality requires skilled technician.
- Arthrography: Diagnosing rotator cuff injury, frozen shoulder (it may even be therapeutic)

Lab Studies

- CBC with diff
- Synovial fluid analysis
- ESR
- CRP
- CPK

(continued)

TABLE 3-3: Diagnostic Approaches (Continued)
Other Studies
• NCS
• EMG
• Cervical myelogram: Can be performed at 6 weeks in patients with a neurologic deficit due to a scapular injury.
AP—Anterior-posterior; CBC—Complete blood count; CRP—C-Reactive protein; CPK—Creatine phosphokinase; EMG—Electromyogram; ESR—Erythrocyte sedimentation rate; NCS—Norcholesterol scintigraphy; MRI—Magnetic resonance imaging.

TABLE 3–4: Common Conditions and Management

A. Acromioclavicular Injury

- **Clinical:** Patient holds his/her arm close to the chest and resists rotation and elevation Anterior shoulder pain or grinding; may have "popping" with reaching overhead and across the chest.

- **Adduction Part of Apley's Test:** Positive

- **Cross Arm Test:** Positive

- **Acromioclavicular Injury Staging (Type I–VI):**

Type I: Sprain, pain and tenderness, normal radiograph
Type II: AC joint widening on radiograph, normal CC joint
Type III: Complete displacement of the clavicle, increase in CC joint space.
Type IV: Superior displacement of the clavicle on AP radiograph and posterior displacement on axillary view.
Type V: CC joint interspace over 100%
Type VI: Distal end of clavicle to lie either in subacromial or subcoracoid space

Source with permission: Rockwood CA Jr. Subluxation and dislocations about the shoulder. In: Rockwood CA Jr, Green DP, eds: *Rockwood and Green's Fractures in Adults*. 3rd ed. Philadephia, PA: JB Lippincott; 1998.

- **Management:** Type I and II: Wear a sling for 5–7 days until pain is relieved

  - 1st 48 hrs → Ice 10–15 min every 6 hrs

  - Analgesics useful for severe pain

  - Return to normal activity and sport within 4 wks

Type III: Treat nonsurgically (as Type I and II) and surgically
Type IV–VI: Treat surgically

B. Adhesive Capsulitis: Also known as frozen shoulder

- **Clinical:** Commonly in patient with diabetes, stroke, parkinsonism, chronic pulmonary disease

(continued)

TABLE 3–4: Common Conditions and Management (Continued)
Commonly secondary from rotator cuff tendonitis
Stiff glenohumeral joint with significant loss of range of motion
• **Management:** NSAIDs/narcotic analgesics
• Moist heat prior to stretching
• Stretching exercises
• Intra-articular corticosteroid injection
• TENS
C. Bicep Tendinitis: Inflammation of long head of bicep tendon as it passes through the bicipital groove of the anterior proximal humerus
• **Clinical:**
• Anterior shoulder pain
• Common with repetitive lifting
• If patient has a *lump* just above antecubital fossa, then it is suggestive of bicep tendon rupture
• Yergason test: Positive
• Speed's maneuver: Positive
• **Management:** Majority of bicep ruptures are treated nonsurgically
• NSAIDs
• Avoid activities that exacerbate the symptoms
• Corticosteroid injections
• Strengthening exercise
D. Bicep Tendon Rupture: Inflammation of long head of bicep tendon as it passes through the bicipital groove of the anterior proximal humerus

(continued)

TABLE 3–4: Common Conditions and Management (Continued)
• **Clinical:**
• If patient has a *lump* just above antecubital fossa, then it is suggestive of bicep tendon rupture.
• **Management:** Partial tears of bicep ruptures are treated nonsurgically
• Ice
• NSAIDs
• Avoid activities that exacerbate the symptoms
• Corticosteroid injections
• Flexibility and strengthening exercise
• **Complete tear:** May require surgical repair
E. Clavicle Fracture
• **Classification:**
(1) Proximal 1/3
(2) Middle 1/3
(3) Distal 1/3
Type I. Nondisplaced, intact CC ligament
Type II. Displaced, CC ligament tear
Type III. Nondisplaced, AC
• **Etiology:** Commonly occurs from a fall onto an outstretched or fall directly onto the shoulder.
• **Clinical:** Watch out for injury to subclavian vessels, manifesting as hematoma, bruit over the region, absent/altered pulses in extremity, first rib fracture, brachial plexus injury, or a wide mediastinum on chest x-ray.

(continued)

TABLE 3–4: Common Conditions and Management (Continued)

- **Management:** Majority of clavicular fractures can be treated nonsurgically with a standard arm sling or a figure "8" clavicle strap. 3–4 wks in child <12 yrs of age and 4–6 wks in >12 yrs of age.

  - **Surgical Treatment:** For open fractures, fracture with neurovascular compromise, concurrent injury to chest leading to rib fracture or flail chest.

F. Glenohumeral Osteoarthritis

- **Etiology:** Secondary from *wear* and *tear* of articular cartilage of the glenoid, labrum, and humeral head

- **Clinical:** Pain, loss of motion in shoulder

- **Management:** Consider NSAIDs

- Heat/ice

- Glucosamine chondroitin sulfate (efficacy not yet proven)

- Corticosteroid injection

- Hyaluronic injection

- Hemiarthroplasty or total joint replacement

G. Humerus Fracture: Neer classification

- **Clinical:** Pain, loss of function with swelling of the involved extremity; may have paresthesias or weakness, or ecchymosis

Fracture fragments	Neer classification
2 part	Anatomic neck fracture
2 part	Surgical neck fracture
3 part	Greater tuberosity fracture
3 part	Lesser tuberosity fracture

Source with permission: Neer CS. Displaced proximal humeral fractures: I. Classification and evaluation. J *Bone Joint Surg Am.* 1970;52:1077–1089.

Management:

- Displacement <1cm fractures: Sling, exercise program after 1 wk

(continued)

TABLE 3–4: Common Conditions and Management (Continued)
• Two part fracture involving greater tuberosity with separation >1cm: Surgical repair
• Two part fracture involving humeral neck: Surgical repair
• Three and four part displaced fracture: Surgical repair
• Four part fracture, which disrupts the vascular supply to the humeral head: Majority of cases requires prosthetic replacement of the proximal humerus.
H. Labral Tear
• **Etiology:** Occurs with high risk athletic activities (baseball pitching, tennis, swimming, golfing, weightlifting).
• **Clinical:** Patient presents with deep shoulder pain, catching sensation, instability, or crepitus
• **Management:** Ice, pain or anti-inflammatory medication, stretching, and strengthening exercises; surgery if unstable joint.
I. Referred Pain to Shoulder
• **Etiology:** Neural impingement at cervical spine due to disc herniation
• Peripheral nerve entrapment distal to spinal column (long thoracic and suprascapular nerve)
• Diaphragmatic irritation (lung disease such as pneumonia, pneumothorax)
• Myocardial infarction
• Abdominal diseases (pancreatitis, cholecystitis)
• Herpes zoster
• **Management:** Treat underlying cause
J. Rotator Cuff Injuries are Categorized into Following:
• **Anatomy:** Rotator cuff consists of supraspinatus, infraspinatus, subscapularis, and teres minor.

(continued)

TABLE 3–4: Common Conditions and Management (Continued)

1. **Impingement Syndrome:** Signs and symptoms resulting from compression of the rotator cuff tendon and the subacromial bursa between the greater tubercle of the humeral head and the lateral edge of acromion process.

   - **Clinical:** Pain and weakness of joint.

   - **Neer Test:** Testing for supraspinatus tendon impingement.

   - **Hawkins Test:** Testing for supraspinatus tendon impingement.

   - **Management:**

     - NSAIDs

     - Avoid activities that exacerbate the symptoms

     - Stretching exercises

     - Corticosteroid injection

     - Strengthening exercises

2. **Rotator Cuff Tendonitis:** Inflammation of supraspinatus (abduction) and infraspinatus (external rotation)

   - **Etiology:** Most commonly occurs with repetitive activity

     - Patient has pain with pushing, pulling, lifting, and reaching the arm above the shoulder.

   - **Clinical:** Patient usually has a pain with lying on the affected shoulder.

     - Stage I: Sore shoulder syndrome

     - Stage II: Profound pathologic pain

   - **Empty can test:** Testing for supraspinatus, infraspinatus, teres minor muscle testing integrity.

   - **Management:**

     - Avoid activities that exacerbate the symptoms

     - NSAIDs

     - Rehabilitation of the rotator cuff

     - Strengthening exercises

(continued)

TABLE 3–4: Common Conditions and Management (Continued)

3. Rotator Cuff Tear: Loss of integrity of rotator cuff

- **Etiology:** Secondary following conditions
  - Injury—fall onto outstretch arm or shoulder, severe pulling or pushing
  - Chronic subacromial impingement
  - Progressive tendon degeneration
- **Clinical:** Pain often over anterolateral shoulder, exacerbated by overhead activites; may have nocturnal pain especially when lying on affected shoulder; weakness, loss of shoulder motion.
  - **Empty Can Test:** For supraspinatus, infraspinatus, teres minor muscle testing integrity
  - **Drop-Arm Test:** for rotator cuff tear or supraspinatus dysfunction
  - **Lift-Off Test:** For supraspinatus muscle function
  - **Sulcus Test:** For inferior glenohumeral instability
  - **Apprehension Test:** For anterior shoulder instability
  - **Relocation Test:** For anterior glenohumeral instability
  - **Apley Scratch Test:** For rotator cuff problem
- **Management:** NSAIDs
  - Avoid activities that exacerbate the symptoms
  - Stretching and strengthening exercises
  - Corticosteroid injection

K. Scapular Instability

- Abnormal shoulder motion or mild scapular winging
- Nerve injury may also lead to winging scapula
- **Clinical:** Abnormal shoulder motion or mild scapular winging. Nerve injury may lead to winging scapula.
- **Management:** Activity modification, strengthening exercises

(continued)

TABLE 3–4: Common Conditions and Management (Continued)
L. Scapula Fracture
• **Etiology:** Normally, scapula fractures result from high-energy trauma.
• **Clinical:** Swelling, tenderness, crepitus, ecchymosis over scapular region
• **Management of Scapular Fracture:**
• For majority of patient a sling is adequate. An early range of motion as tolerated usually within 1 wk of the injury.
• If scapular body fracture → consider hospital admission due to the risk of pulmonary contusion
M. Subcapsular Bursitis
• **Anatomy:** Occurs from pressure and friction between superior-medial angle of scapula and second and third rib
• **Etiology:** Common etiology: kyphotic posture, poor muscle formation in thin individual, professions that involves repetitive motion of the scapula (assembly worker, drycleaner working with ironing, etc.)
• **Management:** Anti-inflammatory medication, corticosteroid injection, physical therapy (strengthening exercises)
AC—Acromioclavicular; AP—Antero-posterior; CC—Coracoclavicular; NSAIDS—Nonsteroidal anti-inflammatory drug; TENS——Transcutaneous electrical nerve stimulation.

TABLE 3–5: Special Tests

A. Apley Scratch Test

- **Indication:** To assess rotator cuff function

- **Technique:** Have patient touch inferior and superior aspect of opposite scapula

- **Interpretation:** Loss of range of motion = rotator cuff problem

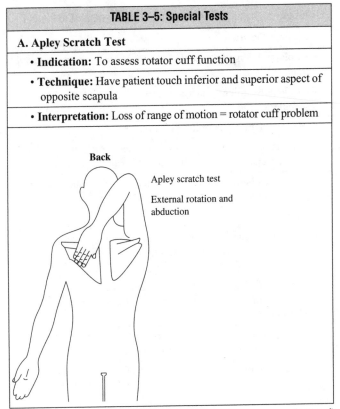

Back

Apley scratch test

External rotation and abduction

(continued)

TABLE 3–5: Special Tests (Continued)

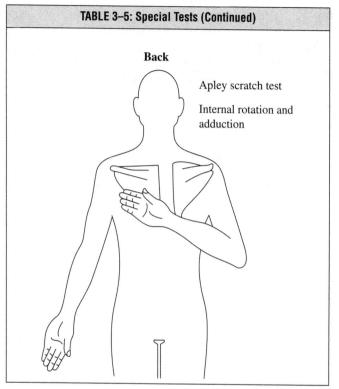

Back

Apley scratch test

Internal rotation and adduction

(continued)

TABLE 3–5: Special Tests (Continued)

B. Apprehension Test

- **Indication:** To assess anterior shoulder instability

- **Technique:** Have patient seated or in supine position, externally rotate the shoulder

- **Interpretation:** Patient resist activity due to fear that shoulder will dislocate = positive

Apprehension test

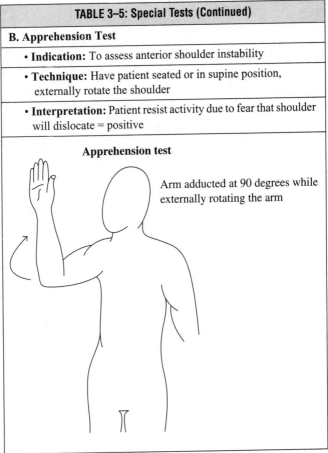

Arm adducted at 90 degrees while externally rotating the arm

(continued)

TABLE 3–5: Special Tests (Continued)

C. Clunk Sign

- Rotation of loaded shoulder from extension to forward flexion. Pain indicates labral disorder.

- **Indication:** To assess labral disorder

- **Technique:** Have patient lie supine, rotate patient's arm with force (loading) from extension to forward flexion

- **Interpretation:** "Clunk" or clicking sensation = labral tear

D. Cross Arm Test

- **Indication:** To assess acromioclavicular joint integrity

- **Technique:** Have patient raise arm to 90 degrees then actively adduct arm

- **Interpretation:** Pain in acromioclavicular joint = positive

Cross arm test

Raising arm to 90 degrees then actively adduct (pain over acromioclavicular joint)

(continued)

TABLE 3–5: Special Tests (Continued)
E. Drop-Arm Test
• **Indication:** To assess for rotator cuff tear or supraspinatus dysfunction.
• **Technique:** Abduct shoulder to 90 degrees then ask patient to lower arm slowly to the side in the same arc of movement
• **Interpretation:** Pain or inability to return arm to the side slowly = positive
F. Empty Can Test
• **Indication:** Rotator cuff injury (supraspinatus muscle testing, infraspinatus, teres minor muscle testing)
• **Technique:** Patient rotate arm with thumbs pointing to the floor while examiner apply resistance with arms in 30 degrees forward flexion & 90 degrees abduction.
• **Interpretation:** Weakness compared to unaffected side = disruption of supraspinatus tendon.
↑ = Patient's force
↓ = Physician's force

(continued)

TABLE 3–5: Special Tests (Continued)

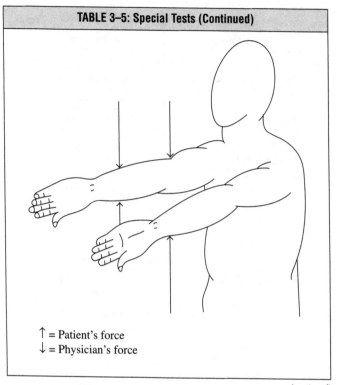

↑ = Patient's force
↓ = Physician's force

(continued)

TABLE 3–5: Special Tests (Continued)	
Internal rotation	**Adduction**
Latissimus dorsi	Latissimus dorsi
Pectoralis major	Pectoralis major
Teres major	Teres major
Deltoid	Coracobrachialis
Subscapularis	Triceps brachii
External rotation	**Abduction**
Deltoid	Deltoid
Infraspinatus	Supraspinatus
Teres minor	Pectoralis major

G. Hawkins Test

- **Indication:** To test for supraspinatus tendon impingement

- **Technique:** Forward flexion of the shoulder to 90 degrees and internal rotation

- **Interpretation:** Pain or grimacing facial expression = impingement

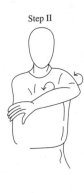

Step I

Step II

Hawkin's test

Testing for supraspinatus tendon impingement

-The arm is forward elevated to 90 degrees then internally rotated

(continued)

TABLE 3–5: Special Tests (Continued)

H. Neer Test

- **Indication:** To test for impingement of supraspinatus tendon

- **Technique:** Forcefully elevate an internally rotated arm in the scapular plane

- **Interpretation:** Pain or grimacing facial expression = impingement

Neer test: Step 1

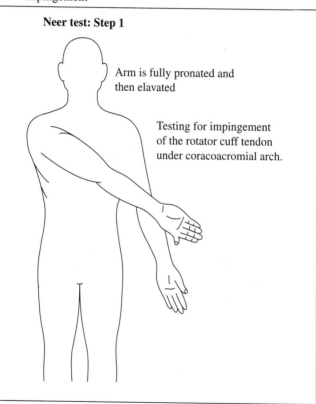

Arm is fully pronated and then elavated

Testing for impingement of the rotator cuff tendon under coracoacromial arch.

(continued)

TABLE 3–5: Special Tests (Continued)

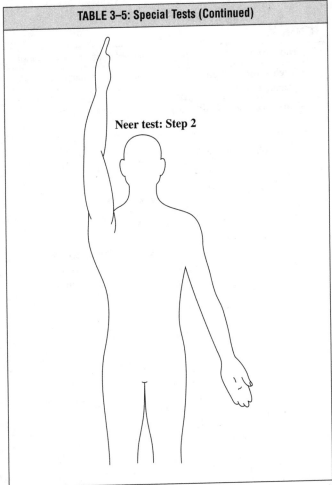

Neer test: Step 2

(continued)

TABLE 3–5: Special Tests (Continued)

I. NFL Touchdown Sign

- **Indication:** To assess shoulder range of motion and abduction

- **Technique:** Ask patient to raise both arms directly overhead

- **Interpretation:** Compare both sides with regards to smoothness of movement, discomfort, completeness of maneuver

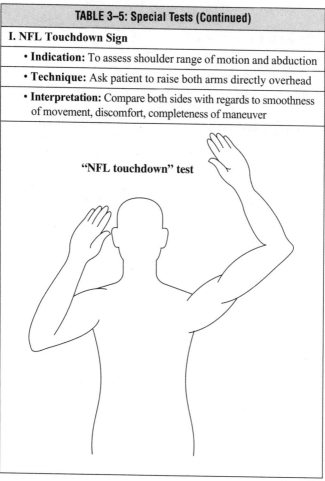

"NFL touchdown" test

(continued)

TABLE 3–5: Special Tests (Continued)

J. Push-Off Test

• **Indication:** To test for subscapularis muscle injury

• **Technique:** Have patient place his/her hand behind his/her back at waist level with palm facing out, then have him/her move the arm from body against your resistance

• **Interpretation:** Pain or inability to move arm from body = positive

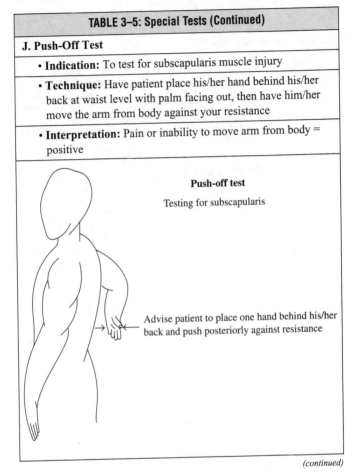

Push-off test

Testing for subscapularis

Advise patient to place one hand behind his/her back and push posteriorly against resistance

(continued)

TABLE 3–5: Special Tests (Continued)

K. Relocation Test

- **Indication:** To assess anterior glenohumeral instability

- **Technique:** Apply posterior force on the anterior proximal humerus while extending the patient's arm further back and release pressure on joint. externally rotating the arm.

- **Interpretation:** Patient becomes anxious and internally rotate the shoulder = anterior glenohumeral instability

L. Speed's Maneuver: Elbow flexed at 20–30 degrees and forearm supinated. Pain indicates bicep tendon instability or tendinitis

- **Indication:** To assess bicep tendon instability

- **Technique:** Flex elbow at 20–30 degrees then supinate forearm

- **Interpretation:** Pain = bicep tendon instability or tendonitis

M. Spurling Test

- **Indication:** To test for cervical root disorder

- **Technique:** While neck extended and laterally rotated, place axial load on spine

- **Interpretation:** Pain = cervical root disorder

Spurling test

Testing for cervical root disorders

The neck is extended and rotated laterally while and axial load is placed on spine

(continued)

TABLE 3–5: Special Tests (Continued)

N. Subacromial Impingement

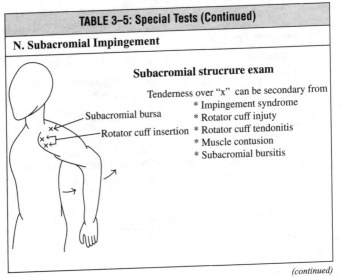

Subacromial strucrure exam

Tenderness over "x" can be secondary from
* Impingement syndrome
* Rotator cuff injuty
* Rotator cuff tendonitis
* Muscle contusion
* Subacromial bursitis

Subacromial bursa

Rotator cuff insertion

(continued)

TABLE 3–5: Special Tests (Continued)
O. Sulcus Test
• **Indication:** To test for inferior glenohumeral instability
• **Technique:** Have patient hold arm in resting position at his/ her side, then pull the arm downward from the elbow or wrist
• **Interpretation:** Depression below the shoulder = positive sign

Sulcus test

Testing for inferior
glenohumeral instability

Patient's arm relaxed in neutral
position, physician pulls patients
hand downward at elbow joint

(continued)

TABLE 3–5: Special Tests (Continued)

P. Yergason Test

• **Indication:** Assess biceps tendon integrity

• **Technique:** Have patient's elbow flexed at 90 degrees with thumb facing upward, then grasp the wrist and resist patient's attempt to supinate and flex at elbow

• **Interpretation:** Pain = biceps tendonitis

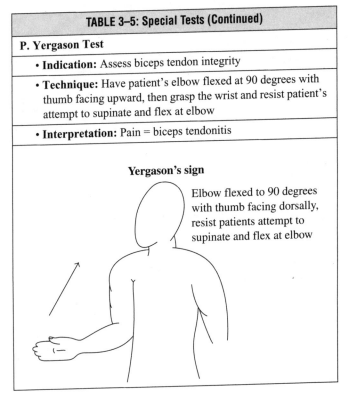

Yergason's sign

Elbow flexed to 90 degrees with thumb facing dorsally, resist patients attempt to supinate and flex at elbow

4
Elbow

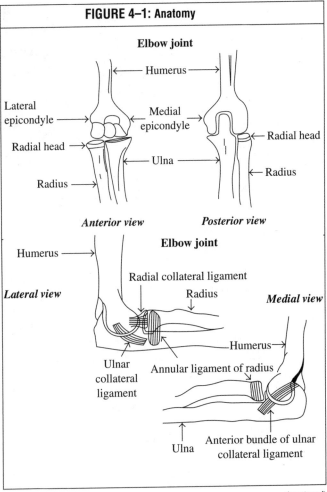

FIGURE 4–1: Anatomy

Elbow joint

Humerus

Lateral epicondyle

Medial epicondyle

Radial head

Radial head

Radius

Ulna

Radius

Anterior view

Posterior view

Elbow joint

Lateral view

Humerus

Radial collateral ligament

Radius

Medial view

Humerus

Ulnar collateral ligament

Annular ligament of radius

Anterior bundle of ulnar collateral ligament

Ulna

(continued)

FIGURE 4–1: Anatomy (Continued)

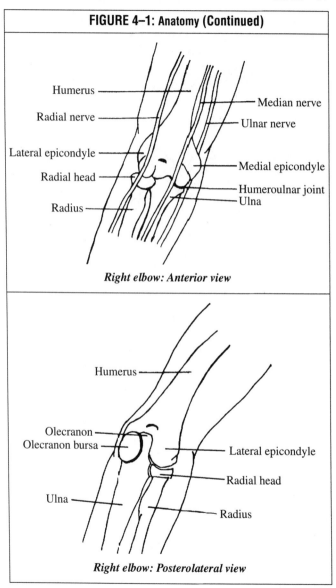

Right elbow: Anterior view

Right elbow: Posterolateral view

(continued)

FIGURE 4–1: Anatomy (Continued)

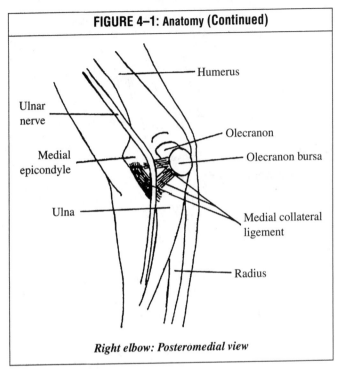

Right elbow: Posteromedial view

TABLE 4–1: Assessment of Injury
A. Inspection: Swelling, erythema, discoloration, deformity, laceration
B. Palpation: Bones and soft tissue—tenderness, deformity, effusion
C. Range of motion: Passive and active
D. Motor
E. Sensory

Elbow Joint Muscle Actions	
Elbow joint action	**Muscles (innervation)**
Flexion	Biceps (musculocutaneous nerve) Brachialis (musculocutaneous nerve) Brachioradialis (radial nerve)
Extension	Triceps (radial nerve) Anconeus (radial nerve)
Pronation	Pronator teres (median nerve) Pronator quadratus (median nerve) Flexor carpi radialis (median nerve)
Supination	Biceps (musculocutaneous nerve) Brachioradialis (musculocutaneous nerve)

• **Motor** (see Chapter 1)
• **Sensory** (see Chapter 1, dermatomal map)
• **Deep tendon reflex** (see Chapter 1)
• **Vascular** (check distal pulses)

TABLE 4–2: Localization of Pain	
Elbow pain	**Differentials**
Anterior	Bicep tendinitis Pronator syndrome Anterior capsule strain
Posterior	Triceps tendonitis Olecranon impingement Olecranon stress fracture Olecranon bursitis
Medial	Medial epicondylitis (Golfer's elbow) Ulnar collateral ligament sprain Ulnar nerve entrapment
Lateral	Lateral epicondylitis (tennis elbow) Radial tunnel syndrome Radiocapitellar chondromalacia Posterolateral rotatory instability
With swelling	Trauma Gout/pseudogout Septic arthritis
Others	Nursemaid's elbow Cervical radiculopathy (neuropathic pain) Osteoarthritis

TABLE 4–3: Diagnostic Approaches		
Imaging studies	**Lab studies**	**Other studies**
• X-ray (AP & lateral)	• CBC with diff	• EMG
• MRI	• Blood C&S	• NCS
	• Synovial fluid analysis	
	• Rheumatoid factor	
AP—Antero-posterior; CBC—Complete blood count; ECS—Electromyogram; NCS—Nerve conduction studies; MRI—Magnetic resonance imaging.		

TABLE 4–4: Common Conditions and Management

A. Elbow Dislocation

Etiology: Usually occurs after trauma. Posterior dislocation is more common than anterior. Most common at ulnohumeral joint.

Clinical: Most common presentation is pain, swelling, deformity, and inability to move the elbow joint.

Management: If neurovascular compromise is detected surgical treatment is required.

B. Lateral Epicondylitis

Etiology: Inflammation of lateral (extensor carpi radialis brevis and longus tendons) epicondyle.

Clinical: Pain exacerbated by wrist extension and radial deviation or supination against resistance and strong gripping or flexing elbow at 90 degrees and then pronating the arm.

Management: Rest, anti-inflammatory medication, immobilization, corticosteroid injection

C. Ligamentous Injury

Etiology: Commonly associated with sports mainly the one that involves throwing an object. Most commonly involved ligament is the medial collateral ligament.

D. Medial Epicondylitis

Etiology: Inflammation of medial (flexor carpi radialis tendon) epicondyle

Clinical: Pain exacerbated by pronating the forearm and flexing the wrist against resistance

Management: Rest, anti-inflammatory medication, immobilization, corticosteroid injection

(continued)

TABLE 4–4: Common Conditions (Continued)

E. Nerve Entrapment

There are three main nerves that pass through the elbow joint. They are as below. They may cause motor and sensory loss/paresthesia in the hand.

(1) Radial nerve entrapment (see Chapter 5)

(2) Median nerve entrapment (see Chapter 5)

(3) Ulnar nerve entrapment (see Chapter 5)

(4) Posterior osseous nerve entrapment syndrome

Clinical: Presents with pain on the lateral side of the elbow, over the area of the muscles of the lateral forearm, distal to the lateral epicondyle of the elbow joint.

• Pain worsened by supination of the forearm.

Management: Rest, splint, surgery

F. Nursemaid's Elbow

Etiology: Occurs from injury to annular ligament, which surrounds the radial head.

• Common after traction injury, such as pulling.

Clinical: Usually presents as mild to moderate pain on palpation, no swelling, and struggle to use the elbow.

Management: Reduction of the displaced annular ligament can be performed by flexing the elbow maximally to the shoulder while supinating the forearm. A "pop" is usually felt during the process.

G. Olecranon Bursitis

Etiology: May be secondary from gout, rheumatoid arthritis, infection, or trauma

Clinical: Swelling over posterior olecranon process, may have normal range of motion.

Management: Bursal aspiration, anti-inflammatory, corticosteroid injection, compressive elbow sleeve.

(continued)

TABLE 4–4: Common Conditions (Continued)	

H. Osteoarthritis

Etiology: Due to elbow being non–weight bearing joint, degenerative processes are rare. Osteoarthritis in the elbow joint can be secondary from intra-articular fracture, avulsion injury to the humeral condyle, or osteonecrosis.

Clinical: Patient may present with pain with extremes of motion. Greater pain with extension than flexion. Severe arthritis can lead to pain with any range motion.

Management: Anti-inflammatory, physical therapy

I. Activities Commonly Associated with Overuse Elbow

Bowling	Biceps tendonitis
Boxing	Triceps tendonitis
Basketball/football/wrestling	Olecranon bursitis
Golf	Medial epicondylitis, radial tunnel syndrome
Gymnastics	Biceps tendonitis, triceps tendonitis
Sport involving throwing an object (Baseball, tennis etc.)	Triceps tendonitis, olecranon impingement, medial epicondylitis, ulnar nerve entrapment
Racquet sport	Triceps tendonitis, lateral epicondylitis, medial epicondylitis, radial nerve entrapment
Rowing	Radial tunnel syndrome
Tennis	Lateral epicondylitis, radial nerve palsy
Weightlifting	Bicep tendonitis, triceps tendonitis, radial tunnel syndrome, ulnar nerve entrapment, radial nerve entrapment

TABLE 4–5: Special Tests

A. Varus and Valgus Stress Test

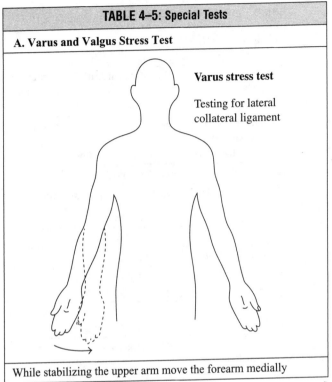

Varus stress test

Testing for lateral collateral ligament

While stabilizing the upper arm move the forearm medially

(continued)

TABLE 4–5: Special Tests (Continued)

Valgus stress test

Testing for ulnar
collateral ligament

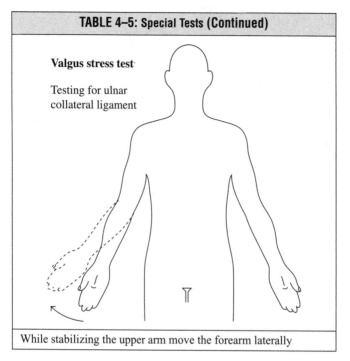

While stabilizing the upper arm move the forearm laterally

FIGURE 5–1: Anatomy

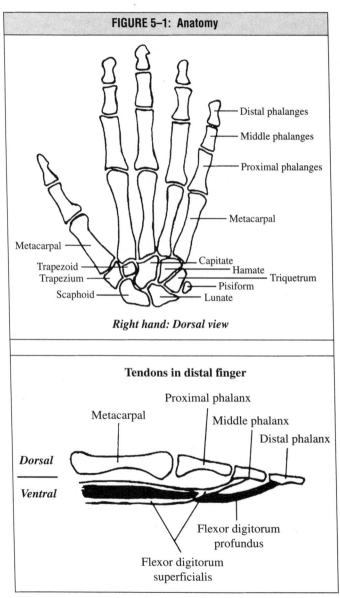

Distal phalanges

Middle phalanges

Proximal phalanges

Metacarpal

Metacarpal

Capitate

Trapezoid

Hamate

Trapezium

Triquetrum

Pisiform

Scaphoid

Lunate

Right hand: Dorsal view

Tendons in distal finger

Proximal phalanx

Middle phalanx

Distal phalanx

Metacarpal

Dorsal

Ventral

Flexor digitorum profundus

Flexor digitorum superficialis

(continued)

FIGURE 5–1: Anatomy (Continued)

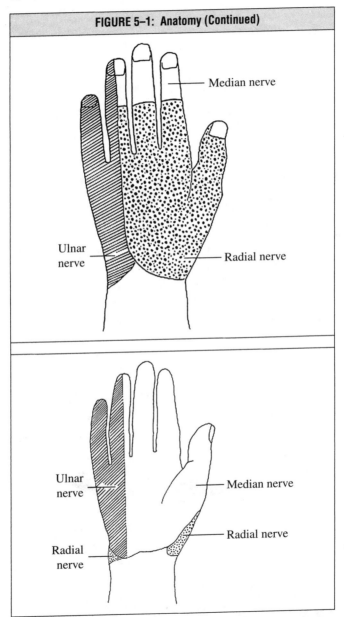

TABLE 5–1: Assessment of Injury

A. Detailed History

B. Inspection: Swelling, erythema, discoloration, deformity, laceration

C. Palpation: Bones and soft tissue—tenderness, deformity, effusion

D. Range of Motion: Passive and active

Wrist	
Flexion	**Extension**
• Flexor carpi radialis	• Extensor carpi radialis longus
• Flexor carpi ulnaris	• Extensor carpi radialis brevis
• Palmaris longus	• Extensor carpi ulnaris
Pronation	**Supination**
• Pronator teres	• Biceps brachii
• Pronator quadratus	• Brachioradialis
• Flexor carpi radialis	• Supinator

Finger	
Flexion	**Extension**
• Flexor digitorum profundis	• Extensor digitorum communis
• Flexor digitorum superficialis	• Extensor digiti minimi
• Lumbricale	• Extensor indices
Abduction	**Adduction**
• Dorsal interossei	• Palmar interossei
• Abductor pollicis brevis	

Thumb (1st) MCP Joint	
Flexion	**Extension**
• Flexor pollicis brevis	• Extensor pollicis brevis
• Flexor pollicis longus	• Extensor pollicis longus

(continued)

TABLE 5–1: Assessment of Injury (Continued)	
Abduction	**Adduction**
• Abductor pollicis brevis	• Adductor pollicis obliquus
• Abductor pollicis longus	• Adductor pollicis transversus
Opposition of Thumb with Little Finger	
• Opponens digiti minimi	
• Opponens pollicis	
Median Nerve Integrity: Opposition of thumb with little finger	
• Motor	
• Sensory	
• Vascular (check distal pulses)	
• Deep tendon reflex	
MCP—Metacarpophalangeal joint	

TABLE 5–2: Localization of Pain
Dorsal Wrist Pain:
Aggravated by flexion/extension
• Ligamentous injury
• Synovium surrounding the joint
• Soft tissue/bony structure injury
Aggravated by movement of the fingers and associated with dorsal swelling
• Tenosynovitis
• Soft tissue/bony structure injury
Pain at the base of the thumb (1st) metacarpal
• May represent carpometacarpal joint osteoarthritis
Dorsal Wrist Swelling
• Ganglion cyst
• Tenosynovitis
• Soft tissue/bony structure injury
Paresthesias, Dorsal Pain, and Hypesthesia (absent or decreased sensitivity to cutaneous stimulation):
• Median nerve compression
• Ulnar nerve compression
Wrist Pain Associated with Weakness with Grip
• De Quervain's tenosynovitis
• Triangular fibrocartilage complex injury
• Hook of hamate fracture
• Carpometacarpal arthritis
• Tendonitis/tendon injury

TABLE 5–3: Diagnostic Approaches
Radiographic Studies:
• X-ray (PA, lateral, oblique)
• CT or bone scan: Useful in diagnosing scaphoid fracture
• MRI
Lab Tests:
• CBC—Evaluation of infectious process
• TSH—Carpal tunnel syndrome (CTS)
• ESR, CRP—Evaluation of inflammatory disease, CTS
• Rheumatoid factor—Rheumatoid arthritis
• Synovial fluid for analysis
• Uric acid—CTS
• Glucose—CTS
Other Tests:
• **Dynometry:** Evaluation of forearm muscle integrity and grip strength
CRP—C-Reactive protein; CTS—Carpal tunnel syndrome; ESR—Erythrocyte sedimentation rate; PA—Posterior-anterior; TSH—thyroid-stimulating hormone

TABLE 5–4: Common Conditions and Management
A. Boutonniere Deformity: Is a result of rupture of the extensor tendon as it inserts into the middle phalanx.
Etiology: It is almost always occurs after trauma.
Clinical: Presents with flexed finger at PIP joint and extension at the DIP joint, painful and tender to touch.
Management: Splint PIP joint for 4–6 wks, surgery may be required if splint does not correct the deformity.
B. Carpal Tunnel Syndrome: Condition leading to neuropathy and motor weakness due to compression of the median nerve.
Etiology: Any condition leading to elevated pressure within the carpal tunnel
(1) Acromegaly
(2) Alcohol
(3) Amyloidosis
(4) Chronic wrist overuse (typing)
(5) Diabetes
(6) Gout
(7) Multiple myeloma
(8) Rheumatoid arthritis
(9) Thyroid myxedema
(10) Trauma
(11) Space occupying lesion within carpal tunnel
Clinical: Sensory changes over median nerve median nerve distribution.
• Chronic condition may have thenar atrophy and wrist weakness.
• Tinel's and Phalen's test—positive
• Durkan carpal compression test—positive

(continued)

TABLE 5–4: Common Conditions and Management (Continued)

Management: Activity modification, cock-up wrist splinting, anti-inflammatory medication, corticosteroid injection, surgical release

C. De Quervain's Tenosynovitis

Clinical: Pain on radial side of thumb and wrist (about 1 cm proximally to radial styloid), may have paresthesia that radiates to thumb, index finger, and dorsum of the hand; palpable swelling
Finkelstein's test: Positive: Pain can be reproduced with having the patient make a fist with the thumb flexed into the palm of the hand and then the wrist is deviated to the ulnar side
Management: Thumb and wrist splint, corticosteroid injection, surgical release

D. Dupuytren Disease: Is a thickening/nodularity and contraction of the palmar fascia

Etiology: Is associated with diabetes, alcoholism, smoking, pulmonary disease, epilepsy, and repetitive trauma
Clinical: May start as nodular lesion, which progresses to a thickening, which eventually leads to contraction and flexion at the metacarpophalangeal joint
• As disease progresses, may involve proximal metacarpophalangeal joint
Management: Splinting, surgery, and occupational therapy

E. Ganglion Cyst: AKA synovial or mucous cyst

• A cystic nodular density arising from a joint capsule or tendon sheath
• Cyst may contain clear to mucinous fluid very similar to joint fluid
• The ganglion is usually smooth, round, and multilobulated

(continued)

TABLE 5–4: Common Conditions and Management (Continued)
Clinical: The lesion may or may not cause pain
• Pain and size may be exacerbated by repetitive movement
• May have sensory and motor defect depending on the location of the cyst
Management: Aspiration, surgical incision and removal
F. Kienböck's Disease: An osteonecrosis of the lunate bone.
Clinical: Pain, stiffness, and swelling over the dorsal aspect of the wrist mainly over the lunate bone.
• Weak grip and inability to grasp heavy objects.
Classification of Lunate Osteonecrosis:
Stage 1   No visible changes noted
Stage 2   Sclerosis of lunate
Stage 3A   Sclerosis and fragmentation of lunate
Stage 3B   Sclerosis and fragmentation of lunate + fixed rotation of the scaphoid or proximal migration of the capitate.
Stage 4   3A or 3B + degenerative changes at adjacent joint
Management: Splint, anti-inflammatory medication
G. Mallet Finger
• Rupture of extensor tendon at the insertion of the base of the distal phalanx
• Avulsion of the distal phalanx injury
Clinical: Presents with pain and failure to straighten the distal phalanx
Management: Splinting of the DIP joint. Avulsion requires surgical repair

(continued)

TABLE 5–4: Common Conditions and Management (Continued)

H. Median Nerve Entrapment

Nerve: C5–T1

Innervation: Pronator teres, flexor carpi radialis, flexor carpi sublimis, flexor pollicis longus, flexor digitorum profundus to 2nd and 3rd fingers, pronator quadratus, abductor pollicis brevis, opponens pollicis, flexor pollicis brevis, 1st and 2nd lumbricals.

Etiology: Trauma, repetitive overuse (flexion, supination, pronation of forearm), compression (fibrous band beneath the pronator teres, or pressure from bicipital bursa)

Clinical: Weakness in wrist pronation, opposition and abduction of the thumb

- Resisted pronation of the forearm and flexion at the wrist joint produces pain over forearm

Management: Rest, splint, anti-inflammatory medication, steroid injection, surgery

I. Metacarpals and Phalanges Fracture

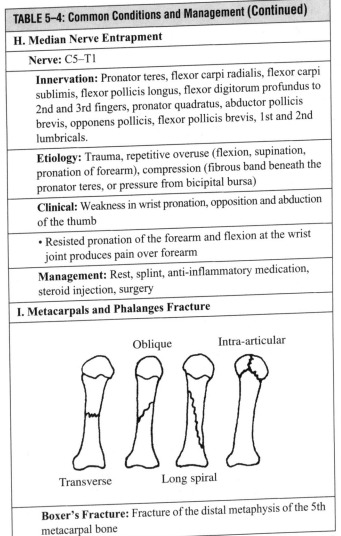

Oblique   Intra-articular

Transverse   Long spiral

Boxer's Fracture: Fracture of the distal metaphysis of the 5th metacarpal bone

(continued)

TABLE 5–4: Common Conditions and Management (Continued)
Metacarpal Fractures
(1) Transverse
(2) Oblique
(3) Spiral
(4) Intra-articular
Phalanx Fracture
(1) Linear
(2) Basal, nondisplaced
(3) Basal, displaced
(4) Comminuted
Clinical: Acute pain and swelling associated with swelling, deformity, and decrease range of motion
Management of Metacarpal Fracture:
• Nondisplaced metacarpal displaced fracture—reduction and immobilization with splint
• Displaced metacarpal neck fracture: Boxer's fracture—ulnar gutter splint
• Stable metacarpal fractures—splinting or casting
• Unstable metacarpal base fracture—operative reduction and fixation
Management of Phalanges Fracture:
• Undisplaced fracture of the diaphysis of the proximal and middle phalanges—buddy taping, casting/splinting
• Undisplaced fracture of PIP joint—buddy taping
• Avulsion fracture of base of proximal phalanx—buddy taping
• Displaced fracture of proximal phalanx—fix with K wire or screws

(continued)

TABLE 5–4: Common Conditions and Management (Continued)
• Displaced diaphyseal fracture—closed reduction
• Displaced unicondylar and bicondylar fracture—open reduction
• Impaction fracture—reduction and fixation
J. Osteoarthritis: AKA degenerative joint disease (DJD)
Clinical: Progressive disease, commonly seen in individuals >40 yrs old
• Due to wear and tear mechanism from overuse of joint, resulting in loss of articular cartilage
• Exacerbated by activity and relieved by rest but advance disease may lead to rest pain
• First carpometacarpal joint is commonly involved and MP joint is not as commonly affected
• Enlargement of the distal interphalangeal joint (DIP): Heberden's node
• Enlargement of the proximal interphalangeal (PIP): Bouchard's node
• Grind test: Positive
Management: Salicylates and anti-inflammatory medications are common mode for pain relief
Intrarticular steroid injection may help
K. Radial Fracture (Distal)
(1) Nondisplaced extra-articular
(2) Nondisplaced intra-articular
(3) Displaced extra-articular
• Dorsally—Colles' fracture
• Volarly—Smith fracture
• Displaced intra-articular

(continued)

TABLE 5–4: Common Conditions and Management (Continued)
• **Universal Classification System:**
Type I: Extra-articular, undisplaced
Type II: Extra-articular, displaced
Type III: Intra-articular, undisplaced
Type IV: Intra-articular, displaced
Clinical: Acute pain associated with swelling and deformity noted at the wrist joint after trauma
Management: Nondisplaced, extra-articular and nondisplaced, intra-articular: short cast, sugar-tongs splint; displaced extra-articular: closed reduction and percutaneous Kirschner-wire fixation with a cast or external fixator or ORIF.
• Open or severely comminuted extra-articular: Closed reduction and percutaneous Kirschner-wire fixation with a cast or external fixator or ORIF
L. Radial Nerve Entrapment
• **Nerve:** C5–T1
• **Above Elbow Entrapment:**
• Innervation: Triceps, anconeus, brachioradialis, extensor carpi radialis longus and brevis
• Defect: Weakness of wrist extension, extension of little finger
• **Below Elbow Entrapment:**
• Innervation: Extensor carpi ulnaris, abductor pollicis longus, finger, and thumb extensors
• Defect: Inability to extend little finger and wrist extension
Clinical: If nerve entrapped above elbow, weakness of wrist and little finger extension
• If nerve entrapped below elbow, inability to extend wrist and little finger
Management: Immobilization (functional splint), anti-inflammatory medication, activity modification, surgical release

(continued)

TABLE 5–4: Common Conditions and Management (Continued)

M. Radial Tunnel Syndrome

Etiology: Trauma, compression (fibrous arcade of Frohse, supinator muscle, bony prominence), congenital anomalous structure

Clinical: Pain and tenderness around lateral epicondyle; may also have "popping" or paresthesia

- Pain elicited by passive resisted extension of the middle finger, resisted forearm supination with elbow extended. Tapping over the radial head may reproduce paresthesia along the course of radial nerve (paresthesia over 4th and 5th fingers) AKA Tinel's sign.

Management: Rest, exercise, and steroid injection

N. Rheumatoid Arthritis

Clinical: Insidious onset of disease; pain, nodular swelling, and stiffness

Criteria: (at least 4 of 7)

(1) Morning stiffness lasting >1 hr

(2) ≥3 joint involvement

(3) Wrist, MCP, or PIP joint involvement for >6 wks

(4) Bilateral/symmetrical joints involvement

(5) Positive rheumatoid factor

(6) Rheumatoid nodule (subcutaneous) over extensor surface

(7) Radiographic evidence of RA

Management: Salicylates and anti-inflammatory medications

- Oral and intrarticular steroid injection may help
- Disease-modifying agents: Hydroxychloroquine, methotrexate, gold

(continued)

TABLE 5–4: Common Conditions and Management (Continued)
O. Scaphoid Fracture: Is the most common fracture on all the carpal bones
Clinical: Mechanism of injury involves axial load to palm with hyperextended wrist
Types:
(1) Distal tubercle fracture
(2) Waist fracture
(3) Proximal-pole fracture
• Localized pain, swelling, and tenderness over radial side of thumb
• Pain also with any wrist motion
• Tenderness over snuffbox
• Scaphoid compression test
• Watson's test
Management: Nondisplaced: ice, elevation, analgesics, thumb spica splint
• Displaced: reduction and fixation with Kirschner wires or screws
P. Tenosynovitis of Extensor Tendon
Etiology: Repetitive activity/overuse
Clinical: Pain over dorsal aspect of the wrist with radiation proximally and/or distally. Pain exacerbated by flexion and extension. Extensor synovial sheath may be palpated
Management: Anti-inflammatory medications, corticosteroid injection

(continued)

TABLE 5–4: Common Conditions and Management (Continued)

Q. Thumb Fracture

- **Bennett's fracture:** A fracture-dislocation of the base of the 1st metacarpal

- **Rolando's fracture:** A comminuted intra-articular fracture of the base of the 1st metacarpal

- **Gamekeeper's thumb:** An avulsion injury of the ulnar collateral of the MCP joint

Clinical: History of trauma with pain, swelling, and tenderness

Management:

- **Bennett's fracture**—Reduced closed under fluoroscopy with stabilization with percutaneous pins

- **Rolando's fracture**—Reduced open through a hockey–stick incision of the volar side of the MCP joint

- **Gamekeeper's thumb**—Open repair of the ulnar collateral ligament and volar capsule through an ulnar incision

- **Extra-articular fracture**—Closed reduction and casting

R. Trigger Finger

Due to thickening or nodular formation over the flexor tendon

Clinical: Painful locking or snapping of MCP or PIP joint

- Difficulty with finger extension after active flexion

- Nodule may be palpated in the palm of hand/finger

Management: Rest, anti-inflammatory medication, lidocaine + corticosteroid injection into tendon sheath, surgical release

S. Ulnar Nerve Entrapment

Nerve: C8–T1

Innervation: Flexor carpi ulnaris, flexor digitorum profundus, palmaris brevis, interossei, lumbricals (3rd and 4th), flexor pollicis brevis

(continued)

TABLE 5–4: Common Conditions and Management (Continued)
Clinical: Inability to abduct little finger
Etiology: Trauma, repetitive movement (flexion and extension at elbow joint), compression (lipoma, ganglion cyst, or tumor)
Management: Elbow pad, rest, splint, anti-inflammatory medication, steroid injection, and surgery
CTS—Carpal tunnel syndrome; DIP—Distal interphalangeal joint; IP—Interphalangeal joint; MCP—Metacarpophalangeal joint; PIP—Proximal interphalangeal; ORIF—Open reduction internal fixation

TABLE 5–5: Special Tests

A. Durkan Carpal Compression Test

Indication: To check for Carpal Tunnel Syndrome (CTS)

Technique: Compress median nerve at wrist for 30 s

Interpretation: Numbness or paresthesia at median nerve distribution (i.e., thumb, index finger and half of middle finger) = positive

B. Finkelstein's Test

Indication: To check for de Quervain's tenosynovitis

Technique: Ulnar deviation to the wrist while grasping the thumb

Interpretation: Pain over radial styloid = de Quervain's tenosynovitis

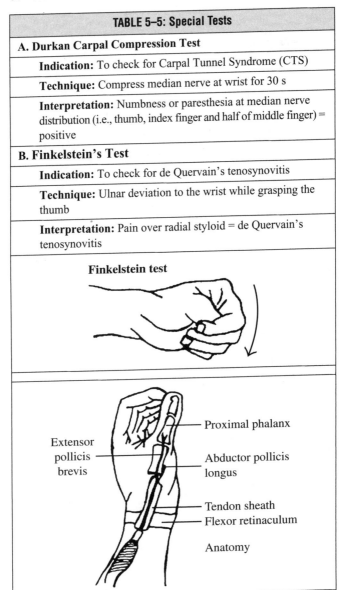

Finkelstein test

Extensor pollicis brevis

Proximal phalanx

Abductor pollicis longus

Tendon sheath

Flexor retinaculum

Anatomy

(continued)

TABLE 5–5: Special Tests (Continued)
C. Froment's Sign
Indication: To assess ulnar nerve palsy specifically test adductor pollicis muscle
Technique: Have patient hold a piece of paper tightly between the thumb and index fingertip while the examiner pulls at the other end of the paper
Interpretation: 1st IP joint flexes to maintain hold on paper = positive for ulnar nerve paralysis and adductor pollicis muscle
D. Grind Test
Indication: To assess for degenerative arthritis or instability
Technique: Compress and rotate the 1st metacarpal bone along the trapezium; compress and rotate the distal radioulnar joint
Interpretation: Pain and crepitus = arthritis or instability
E. Lunotriquetral Shear
Indication: To assess lunotriquetral ligament tear
Technique: Apply dorsal force to triquetrum and palmar force over lunate
Interpretation: Painful click = lunotriquetral ligament tear
F. McMurray's Test
Indication: To assess triangular fibrocartilage complex
Technique: Manipulate the triquetrum against head of ulna with wrist in ulnar deviation
Interpretation: Crepitus, snap, or pain = triangular fibrocartilage complex lesion
G. Phalen's Maneuver
Indication: To reproduce carpal tunnel syndrome
Technique: Flexion of wrist for 30–60 s
Interpretation: Paresthesia over median nerve distribution = CTS

(continued)

TABLE 5–5: Special Tests (Continued)

Phalen's test
This maneuver reproduces carpal
tunnel symptoms

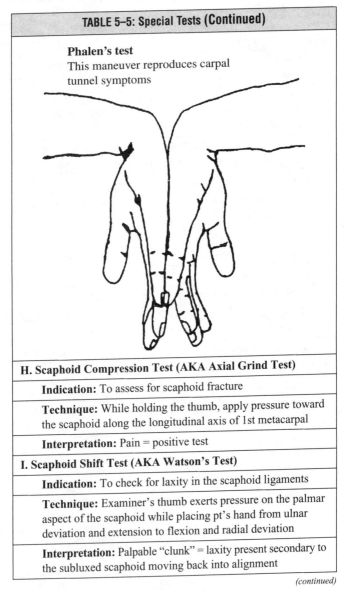

H. Scaphoid Compression Test (AKA Axial Grind Test)

Indication: To assess for scaphoid fracture

Technique: While holding the thumb, apply pressure toward
the scaphoid along the longitudinal axis of 1st metacarpal

Interpretation: Pain = positive test

I. Scaphoid Shift Test (AKA Watson's Test)

Indication: To check for laxity in the scaphoid ligaments

Technique: Examiner's thumb exerts pressure on the palmar
aspect of the scaphoid while placing pt's hand from ulnar
deviation and extension to flexion and radial deviation

Interpretation: Palpable "clunk" = laxity present secondary to
the subluxed scaphoid moving back into alignment

(continued)

TABLE 5–5: Special Tests (Continued)
J. Supination Lift Test: Attempt to lift a heavy object with palms flat under the object, such attempting to lift a table
Indication: To assess triangular fibrocartilage complex
Technique: Have pt lift a heavy object (e.g., table) with palms flat on underside (dorsum of hand facing the floor)
Interpretation: Pain and weakness = triangular fibrocartilage complex injury
K. Tinel's Sign: Tapping on medial nerve reproduces paresthesia over medial nerve distribution
Indication: To reproduce carpal tunnel syndrome
Technique: Performed by tapping the median nerve along its course in the wrist over flexor retinaculum
Interpretation: Paresthesia over medial nerve distribution

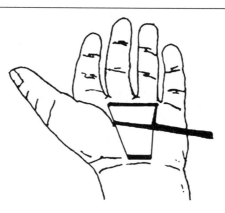

Tinel's test
The maneuver of tapping over the median nerve reproduces carpal tunnel symptoms

(continued)

TABLE 5–5: Special Tests (Continued)
L. Watson's Test
Indication: To assess scaphoid instability or scapholunate separation
Technique: Compress scaphoid tuberosity on palmar aspect while moving the wrist from ulnar to radial deviation
Interpretation: Painful "click" or "pop" = scaphoid instability or scapholunate separation
CTS—Carpal tunnel syndrome; IP—Interphalangeal joint

6
Hip and Thigh

FIGURE 6-1: Anatomy

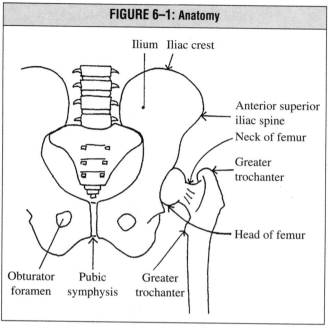

Ilium Iliac crest

Anterior superior
iliac spine

Neck of femur

Greater
trochanter

Head of femur

Obturator
foramen

Pubic
symphysis

Greater
trochanter

(continued)

FIGURE 6–1: Anatomy (Continued)

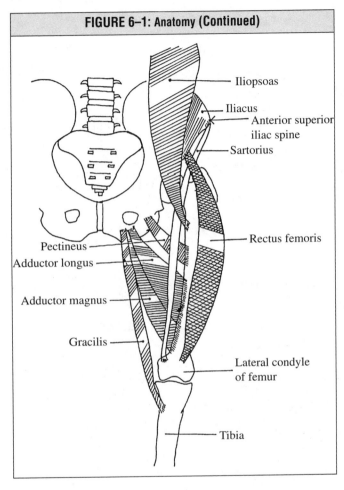

Iliopsoas

Iliacus

Anterior superior iliac spine

Sartorius

Rectus femoris

Pectineus

Adductor longus

Adductor magnus

Gracilis

Lateral condyle of femur

Tibia

TABLE 6–1: Assessment of Injury

A. Detailed History

B. Inspection: Swelling, erythema, discoloration, deformity, laceration, types of shoes

C. Palpation: Bones and soft tissue—tenderness, deformity, effusion

D. Range of Motion: Passive and active

Hip Muscle Actions	
Hip action	**Muscles involved (innervation)**
Flexion	Rectus femoris (also in knee extension; femoral nerve) Psoas (major L1–L2; minor L1) Iliacus (femoral nerve) Sartorius (femoral nerve) Pectineus (femoral nerve)
Extension	Biceps femoris (long head = tibial nerve, short head = common fibular nerve) Gluteus maximus (inferior gluteal nerve) Semimembranous (tibial nerve) Semitendinosus (tibial nerve)
Adduction	Adductor longus (obturator nerve L2–L4) Adductor brevis (obturator nerve) Adductor magnus (obturator and sciatic nerve) Pectineus (femoral nerve) Gracilis (obturator nerve)
Abduction	Gluteus medius (superior gluteal nerve) Gluteus minimus (superior gluteal nerve)
Internal rotation	Gluteus medius (superior gluteal nerve) Gluteus minimus (superior gluteal nerve) Tensor fascia lata (superior gluteal nerve)

(continued)

TABLE 6–1: Assessment of Injury (Continued)

External rotation	Piriformis (nerve to the piriformis)
	Quadratus femoris (nerve to quadratus femoris)
	Obturator internus (nerve to obturator internus)
	Obturator externus (obturator nerve)
	Gluteus maximus (inferior gluteal nerve)
	Gemelli superior (sacral plexus) and inferior (nerve to quadratus femoris)

Hip Muscle Attachment

Muscle	Origin
Sartorius	Anterior superior iliac spine
Rectus femoris	Anterior inferior iliac spine
Iliopsoas	Lesser trochanter
Internal and external oblique	Iliac crest
Hamstring = Biceps femoris (long & short head) + semimembranosus + semitendinosus	Ischial tuberosity (except short head of biceps = linea aspera)

- **Motor** (see Chapter 1)
- **Sensory** (see Chapter 1)
- **Deep tendon reflex** (see Chapter 1)
- **Vascular** (check distal pulses)
- **Gait**

TABLE 6–2: Localization of Pain

Anterior Hip Pain

- Osteoarthritis—Pain and decreased ROM on external rotation and extension
- Muscle and tendon strain
- Tendonitis
- Femoral neck stress fracture—Pain on internal rotation
- Sports hernia (occult hernia or tear of oblique aponeurosis)—Tenderness at superficial inguinal ring
- Obturator or Ilioinguinal nerve entrapment—Adductor tenderness
- Osteitis pubis—Pain on adduction of hip joint, limited rotation
- Acetabular labral tear—Tenderness on internal rotation and extension, click on Thomas test
- Slipped capital femoral epiphysis (Age 12–14 yrs)
- Osteonecrosis

Lower Anterior Hip Pain

- Femur stress fracture (neck)
- Lumbar radiculopathy
- Muscle strain

Lateral Hip Pain

- Trochanteric bursitis—Aggravated by direct pressure
- Fracture
- Meralgia paresthetica—Associated with paresthesia or hypesthesia

Posterior Hip Pain

- Sacroiliac joint pain
- Lumbar radiculopathy
- Piriformis syndrome
- Muscle—strain
- Aortoiliac vascular occlusive disease (Leriche's Dz): may cause thigh pain

ROM—Range of motion

TABLE 6–3: Diagnostic Approaches
Imaging Studies
• **X-ray (Weight-bearing, AP pelvis, Frog leg view)**
This imaging study assesses the following components:
• Pelvic obliquity
• Sacroiliac joints
• Bone density
• Hip joint's articular width (normal is 4–5 mm)
Groin Lateral X-ray
True Lateral
• **Magnetic Resonance Imaging**
MRI is frequently utilized in the following situations:
• Diagnosis and staging of osteonecrosis
• Suspicion of a fracture not seen on a plain x-ray
• Osteomyelitis or other infections
• Tumors
• **Bone Scan**
Radionuclide bone scan is utilized when MRI is not available for the above mentioned situations. The increased activity seen on bone scan is nonspecific and can be caused by a variety of clinical situations such as arthritis, metastatic lesions, fractures, and osteonecrosis.
• **Ultrasonography**
• **Indications:** Guide for effusion aspiration (in adults)
• Hip effusion evaluation (in children)
• Congenital hip dislocation (in infants)

(continued)

TABLE 6–3: Diagnostic Approaches (Continued)

• **Lab Studies:**
• CBC with diff
• ESR, CRP
• Blood C&S
• CPK
AP—Antero-posterior; CBC—Complete blood count; CPK—Creatinine protein kinase; CRP—C-Reactive protein; ESR—Erythrocyte sedimentation rate; MRI—Magnetic resonance imaging

TABLE 6–4: Common Conditions and Management

A. Avascular Necrosis of Hip: Is an osteonecrosis of the femoral head

Etiology: Idiopathic, corticosteroid, ETOH use, hip fracture

Clinical: Presents with acute pain and loss of abduction, internal and external rotation as well as on ambulation

• **Calve-Perthes disease:** Hip avascular necrosis in children, most commonly in the ages between 4 and 12 yrs old

Grading Classifications

Grade	Pain	Physical exam	Radiograph	Bone scan	MRI
0	None	Normal	Normal	Normal	Normal
1	Minimal	↓ internal rotation	Normal	Normal	Some changes
2	Moderate	↓ ROM	Sclerosis	Positive	Positive
3	Severe	↓ ROM	Crescent sign	Positive	Positive
			Femoral head flattening		

(continued)

TABLE 6–4: Common Conditions and Management (Continued)

Management: Core decompression, total joint replacement, anticoagulation
B. Femur Fracture (Proximal)
Etiology: Osteoporosis, trauma, fall
Clinical: Failure to bear weight on leg or ambulate, may have groin pain
• Patient presents with extremity externally rotated, abducted, and shortened
Management: Proximal femoral fracture—Surgery
C. Femoral Neck Stress Fracture
Etiology: Improper training, runner using hard surface, improper footwear
Clinical: Pain at the extremes of passive range of motion, especially external and internal rotation. May have antalgic gait
Management: Rest, ice, elevation, crutches, anti-inflammatory medications, surgery
D. Hip Pointer
Etiology: Direct trauma onto the iliac crest or greater trochanter
Clinical: Tenderness observed over iliac crest. May have pain on ambulation and active abduction
Management: Ice, anti-inflammatory medication, crutches, corticosteroid injection.
• Consult orthopedic surgery if neurovascular compromise.
E. Iliopsoas Tendinitis: Is an inflammation of the iliopsoas tendonitis and surrounding tendon
Etiology: Acute trauma and repetitive hip flexion or external rotation of the thigh
• **Associated sports:** Dancing, ballet, rowing, running, track and field, soccer, gymnastics.

(continued)

TABLE 6–4: Common Conditions and Management (Continued)

Clinical: Insidious anterior hip/groin pain; exacerbated with activity and relieved with rest. Pain may radiate to anterior thigh or knee
• **Ludloff sign:** Pain while sitting with knee extended and elevation of the heel
Management: Physical therapy, anti-inflammatory medications

F. Labral Tear

• **Anatomy:** Glenoid labrum encircles the entire circumference of the glenoid surface. Superiorly, the labrum is adjoined to the tendon insertion of the long head of biceps muscle. The inferior labrum is attached to the glenoid rim.
Etiology: Trauma or fall to the shoulder, athlete using overhead arm (e.g., throwing), gymnastics, weight lifting, idiopathic.
Clinical: Superior labrum anterior posterior (SLAP) lesion – Nonspecific/vague deep shoulder pain, exacerbated with overhead of cross-body activities; commonly presents with "popping," "clicking," or "catching" of the shoulder joint, may also have stiffness or weakness.
• **Superior labrum lesion:** Is a labral detachment/avulsion originating posterior to the long head of the biceps insertion. It is classified into four types.

Superior Labrum Anterior Posterior (SLAP) Classification

I—Degenerative changes and fraying edges noted of the glenoid labrum
No avulsion of the bicep tendon noted
II—Degenerative changes and fraying edges noted of the glenoid labrum
Detachment of the glenoid labrum completely from anterosuperior to posterosuperior rim
Part of labrum is lifted by the long head of the bicep tendon
Bicep tendon is unstable at its attachment on the labrum

(continued)

TABLE 6–4: Common Conditions and Management (Continued)

III—Displacement of free margin of the superior labrum into the joint

Intact labral attachment to the glenoid rim and bicep tendon

Bicep tendon is not unstable at its attachment on the labrum

IV—Displacement of the superior portion of the labrum into the joint with partial rupture of long head of the biceps tendon

Management: Physical therapy, surgery, immobilize with sling, anti-inflammatory medication.

G. Meralgia Paresthetica (AKA Lateral Femoral Cutaneous Nerve Syndrome)

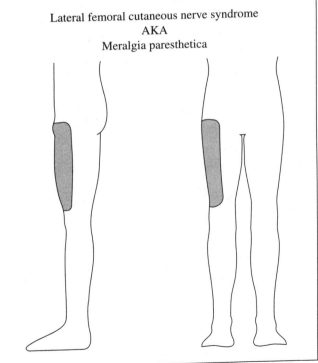

Lateral femoral cutaneous nerve syndrome
AKA
Meralgia paresthetica

(continued)

TABLE 6–4: Common Conditions and Management (Continued)
Etiology: Obesity, tight clothing/belt over the waist, History of surgery over waist, repetitive trauma.
Clinical: Sensory change over distribution of lateral femoral cutaneous nerve pain, burning sensation or paresthesia over anterolateral groin or thigh
Management: Treat the underlying etiology, corticosteroid injection over anterior superior iliac spine, surgical treatment rarely required.
H. Muscle Strain: Iliopsoas strain, hamstring strain, adductor strain
Management: Relative rest, ice, pain management
I. Pelvis Fracture: Fracture of the pelvic ring and/or fracture of the acetabulum
Clinical: Pain over groin area with inability to bear weight, lateral hip or buttocks pain. Pain or range of motion of the hip and on straight leg raising (SLR)
Management: Pain management, physical therapy for gait training, surgical repair
J. Piriformis Syndrome
Clinical: Pain is presented over the buttocks, may radiate to lower leg
• Worse with walking or squatting and intolerance to sitting
• Pain on hip flexion, adduction and internal rotation and palpation of sciatic notch
• **Lasègue sign:** Pain over the greater sciatic notch with knee extension while hip flexed at 90 degrees
• **Pace sign:** Pain and weakness noted with resisted abduction–external rotation thigh
• **Freiberg sign:** Pain noted with passive internal rotation of the extended thigh
Management: Anti-inflammatory medications, physical therapy, local anesthetics, surgery

(continued)

TABLE 6–4: Common Conditions and Management (Continued)

K. Osteoarthritis of the Hip: It is a loss of articular cartilage.

Clinical: Gradual onset of anterior thigh or groin pain, pain may radiate to distal thigh.

- Pain may start with activity and then progress to pain at rest. Stiffness and pain with internal and or external rotation of the hip, limited ROM.

- On this imaging study the following findings are consistent with osteoarthritis:

  (1) Formation of osteophytes (little points of bone growing out)

  (2) Sclerosis(bone along the joint will appear whiter than the surrounding areas)

  (3) Joint space narrowing (bones will be closer than they normally are)

Management: Acetaminophen, anti-inflammatory medication, non–weight-bearing exercise, corticosteroid injection in the affected joint, hip replacement.

L. Slipped Capital Femoral Epiphysis: Displacement of the femoral head and outward rotation of the lower femur

Etiology: Obesity, hypothyroidism, panhypopituitarism, hypogonadism, osteodystrophy

Clinical: Common in ages between 10 and 16 yrs old. Male > female.

- Pain and limited internal rotation or abduction.

- Patient prefers to be in external rotation. Patient may have shortening of leg length.

- Positive Trendelenburg's sign.

Management: Surgery to close physis

M. Trochanteric Bursitis: Inflammation of the bursa superficial to the greater trochanter

(continued)

TABLE 6–4: Common Conditions and Management (Continued)
Etiology: Trauma, idiopathic
Clinical: Pain on palpation of greater trochanter, pain may radiate to the lateral aspect of the thigh. Lateral hip pain can be exacerbated by flexion and abduction of the hip
Management: Relative rest, ice, anti-inflammatory medication, corticosteroid injection

TABLE 6–5: Special Tests
Faber or patrick test Testing for hip and sacroiliac pathology Anterior pain = Hip involvement Posterior pain = Sacroiliac involvement 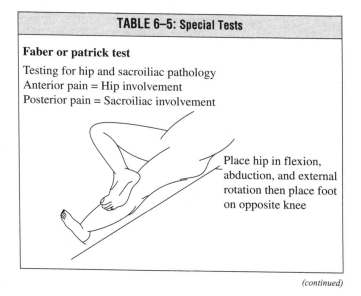 Place hip in flexion, abduction, and external rotation then place foot on opposite knee

(continued)

TABLE 6–5: Special Tests (Continued)

Piriformis syndrome
Palpating the sciatic notch during passive internal rotation

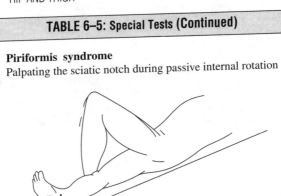

Thomas test
Testing for contractures of hip (Iliopsoas)
and laberal tear

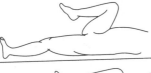

Passive flexion of hip leads
to contralateral leg elevation

30°

Trendelenburg test
Testing for hip abduction. Evaluation of gluteus medius muscle

When patient stands on
one leg, the pelvis will dip
downward due to weak or
nonfunctioning gluteus
medius

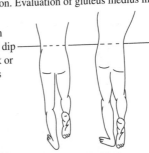

7
Knee

FIGURE 7–1: Anatomy

Anterior view of the knee joint

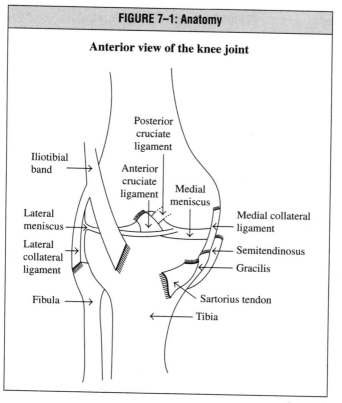

(continued)

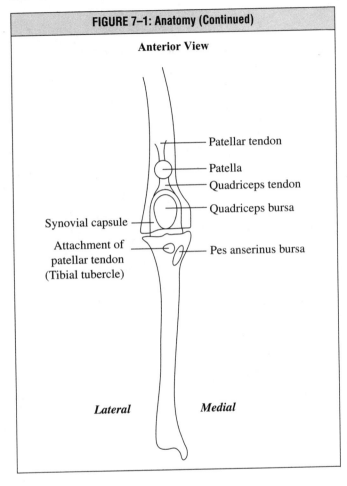

FIGURE 7–1: Anatomy (Continued)

Anterior View

TABLE 7–1: Assessment of Injury	
A. Detailed History	
B. Inspection: Swelling, erythema, discoloration, deformity, laceration	
C. Palpation: Bones and soft tissue—tenderness, deformity, effusion, patellar compression	
D. Range of Motion: Passive and active	
Knee Joint Muscle Actions	
• Flexion	• Extension
• Hamstrings—Semimembranosus	• Quadriceps
• Semitendinosus	• Vastus medialis
• Bicep femoris (long & short head)	• Vastus lateralis
• Gastrocnemius	• Vastus intermedius
• Popliteus	• Rectus femoris
• **Motor** (see Chapter 1)	
• **Sensory** (see Chapter 1)	
• **Deep tendon reflex** (see Chapter 1)	
• **Vascular** (check distal pulses)	
• **Gait**	

TABLE 7–2: Localization of Pain	
Knee Pain	
Anterior	**Posterior**
Patello-femoral syndrome	Popliteal tendonitis
Osgood-Schlatter syndrome	Posterior cruciate ligament injury
Patellar tendonitis	Popliteal cyst
Patellar subluxation	
Patellar dislocation	
Patellar fracture	
Prepatellar bursitis	
Medial	**Lateral**
Patello-femoral syndrome	Iliotibial band syndrome
Medial collateral ligament injury	Popliteal tendonitis
Medial meniscal injury	Lateral collateral ligament injury
Medial plica syndrome	Lateral meniscal injury
Pes anserine bursitis	Lateral compartment osteoarthritis
Medial compartment osteoarthritis	Bicep femoris tendinopathy
Tibial plateau fracture	Degenerative joint disease
	Myofascial pain
	Patellofemoral stress syndrome
	Popliteal tendinopathy

(continued)

TABLE 7-2: Localization of Pain (Continued)

Diffuse Pain with Swelling

• Degenerative joint disease

• Rheumatoid arthritis

• Gout/pseudogout

• Septic arthritis

Pain Over Popliteal Fossa

• Due to large acute effusion exerting pressure in the popliteal fossa especially during knee flexion. The quadriceps muscle pushes the fluid posteriorly, pressuring the gastrocnemius, branches of sciatic nerve and vascular structures. This leads to lower extremities edema, sciatica and localized pain.

• Chronic effusion leads to Baker's cyst (a popliteal cyst)

• Due to distention of gastrocnemius-semimembranous bursa

• Palpated with knee extension as painless mobile swelling located on medial popliteal fossa

Knee Crepitus

• Pt describes it as clicking, crepitation, snapping, popping sounds

• Differentials: patellofemoral syndrome osteoarthritis iliotibial band syndrome (popping sound along lateral femoral condyle) meniscal tear

Sound Manifestation from Knee (Clicking, Grinding, Popping, Snapping, Crepitation)

• Nonspecific but can occur in following settings:

  • Osteoarthritis

  • Patellofemoral syndrome

  • Meniscal tear

  • Iliotibial band syndrome (snapping along lateral femoral condyle)

(continued)

TABLE 7–2: Localization of Pain (Continued)
Knee Effusion
• Indicates intra-articular pathology
• Monoarticular—Gout/Pseudogout
• Seronegative spondyloarthropathies (reactive arthritis. Inflammatory Bowel Disease, psoriasis)
• Rheumatoid arthritis
• Connective tissue disease
• Malignancy
• Septic arthritis
• Fracture
• Advanced osteoarthritis
• Baker's cyst
• Hemarthrosis: Bleeding into a joint/joint spaces
• ACL tear
• Meniscal injury
• Medial collateral ligament injury
• Osteochondral fracture
• Patellar dislocation
• Hemophilia
• Anticoagulation
ACL—Anterior cruciate ligament

TABLE 7–3: Diagnostic Approaches
Imaging Studies:
• **X-ray**
• Weight-bearing AP
• Lateral
• Merchant view (bilateral axial): Especially useful with patellofemoral syndrome demonstrates patellar subluxation.
• **MRI**
• **Bone scan**
• **Venous Doppler**
• **Arterial Doppler**
Lab Studies:
• CBC with diff
• Blood C&S
• Lyme titer
• Synovial fluid analysis
• Rheumatoid factor
• ESR, CRP
Other Studies:
• EMG
• NCS
• Compartment pressure measurement
AP—Antero-posterior; CBC—Complete blood count; CRP—C-Reactive protein; EMG—Electromyogram; ESR—Erythrocyte sedimentation rate; NCS—Nerve conduction studies

TABLE 7–4: Common Conditions and Management

A. Anterior Cruciate Ligament Tear

Clinical: Posttrauma with hyperextension or twisting of the knee. Patient reports of "POP."

- Presents as sudden pain and giving way of the knee. Effusion may be present due to bleeding.

Tests: Lachman test (see Table 7–5).

Management: Rest, ice, compression, anti-inflammatory medication, knee brace, elevation of extremity, crutches, surgical repair.

B. Avascular Necrosis of the Femoral Condyle: Is due to loss of the blood supply to that area. Most commonly involved area is the medial femoral condyle.

Etiology: Idiopathic, chronic steroid injections, renal transplant, sickle cell, SLE, and Goucher disease.

Clinical: Sharp sudden pain over the medial compartment. Effusion may be present. Pain is reproduced over the medial compartment on palpation.

Management: Unloading brace, anti-inflammatory medication, strengthening of quadriceps. Surgery if no response to supportive management.

C. Bursitis of the Knee: (Most Common Prepatellar and Pes Anserine)

Clinical: Pain is noticed with activity or prolonged sitting/ resting, may have localized swelling

- Bursitis may get infected and present with warmth, erythematous, and fever

Management: Ice, anti-inflammatory medication, modification of the activities, ultrasound, phonophoresis, corticosteroid injection

- Antibiotic if infection is noted

(continued)

TABLE 7–4: Common Conditions and Management (Continued)		
D. Collateral Ligament Tear (Medial and Lateral)		
Clinical: Localized stiffness, pain, or swelling may be noted over medial or lateral side aspect		
Tests: Valgus and Varus stress tests (see special tests section)		
Grading of collateral ligament injury	**Ligamentous tear**	**Joint laxity**
1	Minimal	None
2	Moderate	Present
3	Complete	Present
Management: Rest, ice, compression, anti-inflammatory medication, knee brace, elevation of extremity, crutches, surgical repair		
• Grade 1 and 2: Treat nonsurgically		
• Grade 3: Treat surgically		
E. Compartment Syndrome		
• Increased intracompartmental pressure that compromises blood flow		
• Lower leg is divided into four compartments		
A. Anterior		
B. Lateral		
C. Deep posterior		
D. Superficial posterior		
Clinical: Pain out of proportion and paresthesia over the dorsal/plantar aspect of the foot, marked swelling, and tenderness		
• Vascular compromise		
• 5Ps: Pain, pallor, paresthesia, poikilothermia, paralysis		
Management: Immediate fasciotomy		

(continued)

TABLE 7–4: Common Conditions and Management (Continued)
F. Distal Femur Fracture
Classification: Extraarticular shaft fracture
• Unicondylar fracture
• Bicondylar or intercondylar fracture
Management: Nondisplaced or minimum displacement: Nonsurgical
• Displaced: Surgical (open reduction internal fixation)
G. Iliotibial Band Syndrome
• Iliotibial band extends from anterior superior iliac spine to lateral tibia at Gerdy's tubercle. Iliotibial band syndrome develops from the friction of ITB with lateral femoral condyle, which leads to inflammation of the band.
• This condition is common in runners and cyclist.
Clinical: Patient may present with pain over anterolateral aspect of the knee. Patient may also have "popping" with ambulation or running.
• Tenderness to palpation over lateral femoral condyle, positive Noble's and Ober's test.
Management: Ice, anti-inflammatory medication, modification of activities, local corticosteroid injection, physical therapy.
H. Medial Gastrocnemius Tear
• The tear occurs at the muscle–tendon junction.
• Commonly seen in individual participating in tennis, running, and jumping.
Clinical: Individuals may feel pulling or tearing sensation and presents with pain, swelling, and tenderness to palpation.
Management: Rest, ice, calf sleeve/brace, elevation and anti-inflammatory medication, crutches followed by exercise program in 7–21 days.

(continued)

TABLE 7–4: Common Conditions and Management (Continued)
I. Meniscal Tear
• There are two meniscus located in the knee: lateral and medial. They work as shock absorbers and are made of fibrocartilaginous pads.
Clinical: History of twisting of the knee with pain over medial or lateral side of the knee; acute onset of pain, swelling, and stiffness followed by locking and catching.
McMurray test: Positive
Management: Rest, ice, compression (knee brace), elevation, and anti-inflammatory medication. Surgical debridement and repair may required with significant damage. Physical therapy and rehab is beneficial as well.
J. Osteoarthritis of the Knee
Criteria: 3/6 should be present
• >50 yrs of age
• Morning stiffness for <30 min
• Crepitus
• Bony tenderness
• Bony enlargement
• No palpable warmth
Diagnosis: Obtaining weight-bearing film in full extension.
Management: Heat, anti-inflammatory medication, acetaminophen, viscosupplementation, corticosteroid intra-articular injection, knee replacement.
K. Osteochondritis Dissecans
• It is an osteonecrosis of subchondral bone. Posterolateral side of the medial femoral condyle is the most common location in the knee. The condition is a result of small stresses to the subchondral bone that disrupt the blood supply to the bone.

(continued)

TABLE 7–4: Common Conditions and Management (Continued)
Clinical: Pain usually presents as gradual and may have knee effusion and locking of the knee. Tenderness is usually present over the involved region.
Wilson test: Positive
Management: If overlying articular cartilage is intact: Avoidance of running and jumping, immobilization, crutches.
• If skeletal maturity has developed, surgery is required.
L. Patella Fracture
Classification: Nondisplaced
• Polar
• Transverse
• Vertical
• Stellate
• Osteochondral
Management: Nondisplaced fracture—nonsurgical
• Displaced fracture—surgical
M. Patellofemoral Pain Syndrome: Is defined as a peripatellar or retropatellar pain due to changes in the patellofemoral joint
Etiology: Idiopathic, overuse, overload, muscular dysfunction, and biomechanical: Pes planus (flat foot)
• Pes cavus (high arched foot)
• Q angle
Clinical: Pain is presented as diffuse, aching, mainly over the anterior knee
• Pain is exacerbated with prolonged sitting, going up the stairs, squatting, or jumping

(continued)

TABLE 7–4: Common Conditions and Management (Continued)
Patella apprehension test: Positive
Management: Rest, anti-inflammatory medication, quadriceps strengthening (PT)
• Weight loss if obese
N. Popliteal Cyst: AKA Baker's or Synovial Cyst.
• Development of the cyst in the popliteal bursa located in the posterior of the knee.
• They are associated with rheumatoid arthritis and degenerative meniscal tears.
Clinical: Swelling and tenderness over the posterior of the knee joint without any history of trauma or fall. May also present with calf pain.
Management: Nonruptured—Treat underlying etiology, aspiration of the fluid from the cyst, excision of the cyst.
• Ruptured cyst: Rest, anti-inflammatory medication, and elevation.
O. Posterior Cruciate Ligament Tear: Extends from medial intercondylar femur to posterior aspects of tibia.
• Common condition that are prone to PCL injury are as follow:
• Dashboard injury
• A fall with flexed knee and plantar flexion of the foot
• Hyperflexion injury
Clinical: Limited range of motion with effusion. Individual may also have pain and feeling of instability.
Posterior drawer sign: Positive (see Table 7–5)
Management: Exercises that emphasize strengthening of the quadriceps
• Knee brace
• Surgical repair

(continued)

TABLE 7–4: Common Conditions and Management (Continued)
P. Quadriceps/Patellar Rupture: Common after trauma to the knee in flexed position.
Clinical: Severe pain and swelling associated with sensation of "giving way" on ambulation. Patient has difficulty extending the knee joint.
Management: Partial rupture: Immobilization, rest, anti-inflammatory medication
• Complete rupture: Surgical repair is warranted.
Q. Quadriceps/Patellar Tendinitis
Anatomy: (A) Quadriceps muscle inserts on superior pole of the patella.
(B) Patellar tendon inserts on inferior pole of the patella and tibial tubercle.
Clinical: A localized point tenderness over the insertion site of the tendon.
• Pain is exacerbated with activity such as going down the stairs, sitting, squatting, running, and climbing; patient have pain with hyperflexion on exam.
Management: Rest with avoidance of activities that exacerbate the pain, knee immobilizer/brace, ice, anti-inflammatory medication followed by physical therapy.
• **Note:** Avoid corticosteroid injection.
R. Plica Syndrome: Is an inflammation of the plica which is a fold of the synovium.
(1) Suprapatellar plica—Extend from the posterior of the quadriceps tendon to the medial/lateral capsule of the knee.
(2) Medial plica—Extends from the medial joint capsule to the medial anterior fat pad.
(3) Infrapatellar plica—Extends anterior and cover the anterior cruciate ligament.

(continued)

TABLE 7–4: Common Conditions and Management (Continued)
Clinical: Acute pain after trauma or fall. Presents with anterior or anteromedial pain.
• May have snapping or popping noise from the knee. May be able to palpate a thickened plica with knee flexed.
Management: Activity modification, anti-inflammatory medication, local anesthetic with corticosteroid injection, Surgery followed by physical therapy.
S. Shin Splints: Is an inflammation of the tibial periosteum from repetitive muscle contraction
Clinical: Presents as gradual onset of the pain over middle—distal third of the medial tibia. Pain is exacerbated by exercise mainly running.
Management: Avoidance of activity, ice, anti-inflammatory medications, calf sleeve/brace, ultrasound with phonophoresis, foot/ankle strengthening exercises
T. Tibial Plateau Fracture
Classification:
• Lateral split
• Lateral split-depression
• Lateral depression
• Medial split
• Medial and lateral split (bicondylar)
• Medial and lateral split with metaphyseal-diaphyseal dissociation
Management:
• Nondisplaced or minimal displaced: Nonsurgical
• Displaced: Surgical (Open Reduction Internal Fixation)

TABLE 7–5: Special Tests

A. Anterior Drawer Test

Indication: To assess anterior cruciate ligament integrity

Technique:

- Flex knee at degrees

- Stabilize foot by sitting on it

- Grasp proximal tibia with both hands then pull forcibly anteriorly

- Note for laxity, pain, abnormal movement, and compare with opposite side

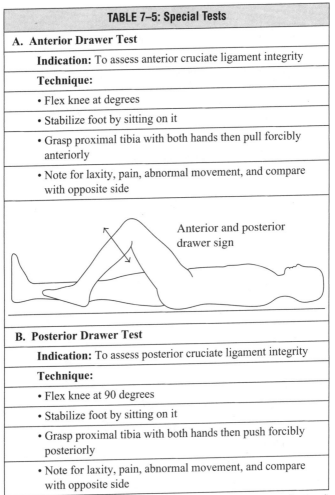

Anterior and posterior drawer sign

B. Posterior Drawer Test

Indication: To assess posterior cruciate ligament integrity

Technique:

- Flex knee at 90 degrees

- Stabilize foot by sitting on it

- Grasp proximal tibia with both hands then push forcibly posteriorly

- Note for laxity, pain, abnormal movement, and compare with opposite side

(continued)

TABLE 7–5: Special Tests (Continued)

C. Lachman Test

Indication: To assess anterior cruciate ligament rupture

Technique:

• Keep knee flexed at 10–20 degrees

• Stabilize distal femur with nondominant hand

• Grasp proximal tibia just below popliteal space

• Place thumb over joint line anterolaterally

• Pull tibia anteriorly and proximally

• Evaluate for end-point laxity

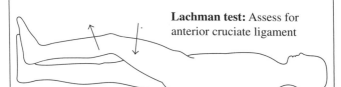

Lachman test: Assess for anterior cruciate ligament

D. McMurray Test

Indication: To assess smooth motion of joint by passive flexion and extension

Technique:

• Place thumb and index finger over medial and lateral joint lines

• Passively flex knee

• Rotate knee medially while applying torque to foot to trap lateral meniscus and then laterally to trap medial meniscus (will note a painful CLICK)

• Passively extend knee

• Repeat step 3 and feel for popping sensation along joint line

(continued)

TABLE 7–5: Special Tests (Continued)

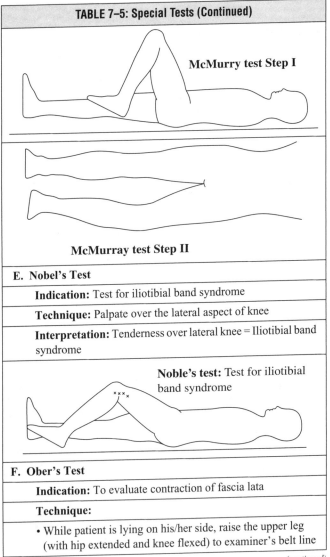

McMurry test Step I

McMurray test Step II

E. Nobel's Test

Indication: Test for iliotibial band syndrome

Technique: Palpate over the lateral aspect of knee

Interpretation: Tenderness over lateral knee = Iliotibial band syndrome

Noble's test: Test for iliotibial band syndrome

F. Ober's Test

Indication: To evaluate contraction of fascia lata

Technique:

• While patient is lying on his/her side, raise the upper leg (with hip extended and knee flexed) to examiner's belt line

(continued)

TABLE 7–5: Special Tests (Continued)
• While supporting the ankle, ask patient to allow leg to drop
• If one feels resistance, means that this is positive Ober's test and may require stretching of the iliotibial band
Interpretation:
• If upper leg reaches a plane at least parallel to the table it is a negative test.

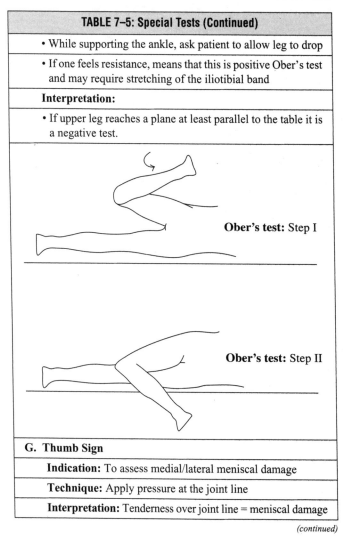

Ober's test: Step I

Ober's test: Step II

G. Thumb Sign
Indication: To assess medial/lateral meniscal damage
Technique: Apply pressure at the joint line
Interpretation: Tenderness over joint line = meniscal damage

(continued)

TABLE 7–5: Special Tests (Continued)

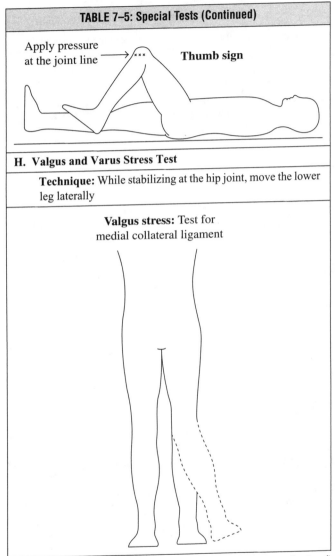

Apply pressure at the joint line → **Thumb sign**

H. Valgus and Varus Stress Test

Technique: While stabilizing at the hip joint, move the lower leg laterally

Valgus stress: Test for medial collateral ligament

(continued)

TABLE 7–5: Special Tests (Continued)

Technique: While stabilizing at the hip joint, move the lower leg medially

Varus stress: Test for
lateral collateral ligament

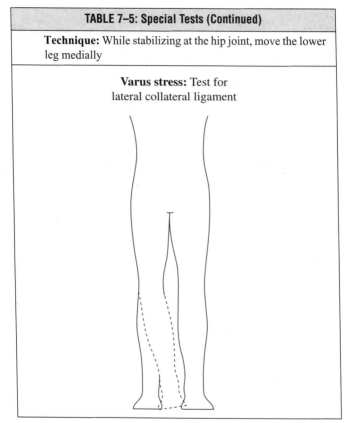

(continued)

TABLE 7–5: Special Tests (Continued)

I. Wilson's Test

Indication: To assess osteochondritis dissecans (OCD)

Technique: With patient supine, flex hip at 90 degrees, internally rotate the tibia then slowly extend the knee.

Interpretation: Pain worse on knee extension to 30 degrees flexion = positive OCD

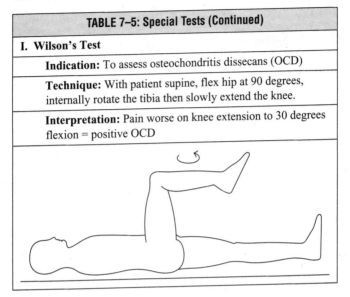

8
Ankle and Foot

FIGURE 8–1: Anatomy

Bones of the Foot

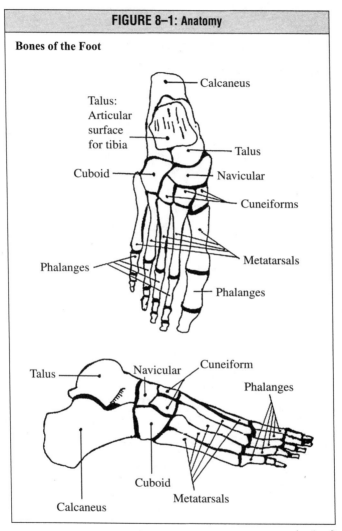

(continued)

FIGURE 8–1: Anatomy (Continued)

Ligaments and Tendons of the Foot

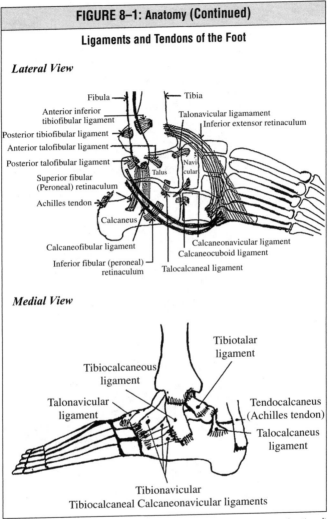

Lateral View

Fibula — Tibia
Anterior inferior tibiofibular ligament
Talonavicular ligamament
Inferior extensor retinaculum
Posterior tibiofibular ligament
Anterior talofibular ligament
Posterior talofibular ligament
Talus   Navicular
Superior fibular (Peroneal) retinaculum
Achilles tendon
Calcaneus
Calcaneofibular ligament
Calcaneonavicular ligament
Calcaneocuboid ligament
Inferior fibular (peroneal) retinaculum
Talocalcaneal ligament

Medial View

Tibiotalar ligament
Tibiocalcaneous ligament
Talonavicular ligament
Tendocalcaneus (Achilles tendon)
Talocalcaneus ligament
Tibionavicular
Tibiocalcaneal Calcaneonavicular ligaments

(continued)

FIGURE 8–1: Anatomy (Continued)

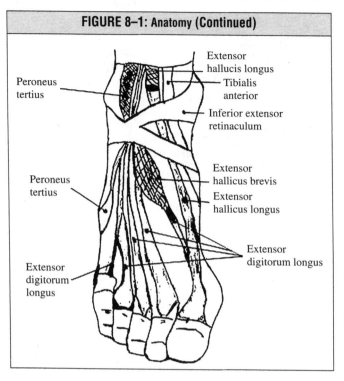

Peroneus tertius

Extensor hallucis longus

Tibialis anterior

Inferior extensor retinaculum

Extensor hallicus brevis

Extensor hallicus longus

Peroneus tertius

Extensor digitorum longus

Extensor digitorum longus

TABLE 8–1: Assessment of Injury

A. Detail History
B. Inspection: Swelling, erythema, discoloration, deformity, laceration, arches, shoes
C. Palpation: Bones and soft tissue—tenderness, deformity, effusion
D. Range of Motion: Passive and active

Ankle Joint

- **Dorsiflexors:** If the peroneal nerve is injured **or** affected in any way from functioning the result is—FOOT DROP
  - **Tibialis anterior:** To test have the patient invert his/her ankles and then ask them to walk on their heels
    - Innervated by deep peroneal nerve, L4
  - **Extensor hallucis longus and extensor digitorum longus:**
    - To test have the patient place their feet in neutral position and then ask them to walk on their heels
    - Innervated by deep peroneal L5
- **Plantar flexors:**
  - **Peroneus longus and brevis:** To test have the patient walk on the medial borders of his/her feet
    - Main function is evertors of the foot and ankle
    - Innervated by superficial peroneal nerve, S1

Gastrocnemius and soleus:

(1) To test ask the patient to walk on his/her toes OR

(2) Have patient jump up and down on the balls of his foot, test is positive for weakness of muscles if patient lands flat-footed. Innervated by tibial nerve, S1, S2

(continued)

TABLE 8–1: Assessment of Injury (Continued)

Flexor hallucis longus:

(1) Observe patient's gait specifically the toe-off phase of the gait

(2) To test stabilize the patient's calcaneus and ask him/her to dorsiflex the great toe and then plantar flex. Resist patient's plantar flexion of great toe. Compare with other side for the relative strength.

Innervated by tibial nerve, L5

Flexor digitorum longus:

- To test stabilize patient's calcaneus, patient then curls his/her toes and physician should resist this flexion.

- Innervated by tibial nerve, L5

- **Tibialis posterior:**

  - To test stabilize patient's foot and ask patient to plantar flex and invert his/her foot and physician should resist this motion

  - Innervated by tibial nerve, L5

- **Adduction:**

Involves primarily the midtarsal joint:

- Calcaneocuboid joint

- Talonavicular joint

- **Abduction:**

Involves primarily the midtarsal joint:

- Calcaneocuboid joint

- Talonavicular joint

- **Eversion**

- Peroneal longus

- Peroneal brevis

- Peroneal tertius

- Ligament support—talofibular and calcaneofibular

(continued)

TABLE 8–1: Assessment of Injury (Continued)
• **Inversion**
• Tibialis anterior
• Tibialis posterior
• **Big toe extension**
• Extensor hallucis longus
Metatarsophalangeal Joint
• **Flexion**
• Flexor digitorum brevis
• Flexor hallucis brevis
• Flexor digitorum brevis
• Flexor hallucis longus
• Flexor digiti minimi brevis
• Flexor digitorum longus
• Interossei
• Lumbricales
• Quadratus plantae
• **Extension**
• Extensor hallucis longus
• Extensor digitorum
• Extensor digitorum brevis
• **Abduction**
• Abductor hallucis
• Abductor digiti minimi
• Dorsal interossei

(continued)

TABLE 8–1: Assessment of Injury (Continued)
Interphalangeal Joint
• **Flexion**
• Flexor hallucis longus
• Flexor digitorum longus
• Flexor digitorum brevis
• Quadratus plantae
• **Extension**
• Extensor hallucis longus
• Extensor digitorum longus
• Extensor digitorum brevis
• **Motor** (see Chapter 1)
Sensory (also see Chapter 1)
• L4: Medial side of foot, medial malleolus
• L5: Dorsum of foot
• S1: Lateral side of foot
• Saphenous nerve: Medial side of foot
• Peroneal nerve: Dorsum of foot
• Sural nerve: Lateral side of foot
Deep tendon reflex (see Chapter 1)
Vascular (check distal pulses)

TABLE 8–2: Localization of Pain		
Pain location	**Differentials**	
Forefoot	• Arthritis • Stress fracture • Gout	• Neuroma • Bursitis
Midfoot and hindfoot	• Stress fracture • Plantar fasciitis • Tendinitis	• Tarsal tunnel syndrome (Pain inferior to medial malleolus on dorsiflexion-eversion)
Heel	• Achilles tendonitis • Tarsal tunnel syndrome • Plantar fasciitis • Heel pad atrophy	• Retrocalcaneal bursitis • Fracture • Retroachilles bursitis
Plantar foot	• Plantar fasciitis • Neuroma • Plantar fascia rupture • Bone cyst	• Heel pad atrophy • Fracture • Tarsal tunnel syndrome • Tumor
Ankle	• Ankle sprain • Achilles tendon rupture • Fracture • Tendon injury • Ligament injury	• Shin splints syndrome • Achilles tendinitis • Stress fracture • Distal tibia-fibula injury • Compartment syndrome
Chronic ankle pain	• Ankle fracture • Peroneal nerve entrapment • Talotibial exostosis	• Peroneal tendon subluxation • Osteochondritis dissecans • Lateral impingement

TABLE 8–3: Diagnostic Approaches

Imaging Studies:
• Ankle: X-ray (AP, lateral, and mortis)
• Foot: X-ray (weight-bearing AP, lateral, and supine oblique)
• MRI
• Bone scan
• Arterial Doppler
Lab Studies:
• CBC with diff
• Blood C&S
• Synovial fluid analysis
• Rheumatoid factor
• ESR, CRP
• CPK
Other studies:
• NCS
• EMG
AP—Antero-posterior; CBC—Complete blood count; CPK—Creatinine protein kinase; CRP—C-Reactive protein; ESR—Erythrocyte sedimentation rate; MRI—Magnetic resonance imaging

TABLE 8–4: Common Conditions and Management

A. Accessory Navicular: It consists of an ossicle, located medial to the navicular bone
It is a normal anatomical variant
Etiology: Nonfitting shoes or trauma
Clinical: Pain can be exacerbated by having pt stand on their feet
• It can be distinct over medial aspect of the navicular bone
Management: Rest, anti-inflammatory medication, proper orthotics
B. Achilles Rupture: Disruption of the Achilles tendon. Its insertion site is calcaneus bone
Etiology: Trauma, chronic Achilles tendinitis, previous partial tear not properly treated
Management: Surgical, cast treatment
C. Achilles Tendinitis: Inflammation of the Achilles tendon and its sheath
Etiology: Overuse especially when associated with hard/uneven surface, improper shoes, extreme cold weather, lack of warm-up prior to activity
Clinical: Pain exacerbated by running/jumping and may increase with dorsiflexion
• Pain over insertion of Achilles tendon on calcaneus
Management: Rest, anti-inflammatory medication, stretching and strengthening, proper footwear.
D. Ankle Arthritis
Etiology: Most commonly secondary from obesity and trauma. Common age >50 yrs
• Usually presents with pain and loss of range of motion
Management: Limit activity, anti-inflammatory medication, proper orthotics

(continued)

TABLE 8–4: Common Conditions and Management (Continued)

E. Ankle Fracture

Etiology: Trauma, fall, or sports injury

- Two classification systems
- Lauge-Hansen classification (extended)
- OA (orthopedic trauma) classification

Clinical: Ecchymosis and swelling is common, unable to bear weight and ankle pain

Management: Pain management, elevation, splint, or cast in a natural position

- If joint widening noted on x-ray: Operative treatment usually is required

F. Ankle Sprain

Ankle Sprain Grading

	Grade 1	Grade 2	Grade 3
Pain	Minimum	Moderate	Severe
Swelling	Minimum	Moderate	Severe
Ecchymosis	None	Frequently	Almost always
Loss of function	Minimum	Moderate	Severe
Tendon	No tear	Partial tear	Complete tear
Difficulty bearing weight	None	Usually	Almost always

Management

Grade 1 → Medical management (rest, ice compression, anti-inflammatory)

Grade 2 → Medical management (rest, ice compression, anti-inflammatory)
  → Casting may be helpful

Grade 3 → Casting vs. surgery

(continued)

TABLE 8–4: Common Conditions and Management (Continued)
G. Compartment Syndrome
Foot consists of nine compartments (1) Medial, (2) Lateral, (3) Central, (4) Calcaneal, (5) Four interossei compartments, (6) Adductor muscle compartment
Etiology: High-energy injury, crush injury
Clinical: Intense pain with severe swelling of the foot after trauma, diminished/absence of pulses
Management: Stat surgical decompression with fasciotomy
H. Freiberg's Disease: An avascular necrosis of the 2nd metatarsal head, rarely it may involve other metatarsals
Clinical: Young individual with pain over 2nd MTP, that is exacerbated with activity and relieved by rest
Management: Avoid exacerbating activites: hard—sole shoe; short—leg walking cast, metatarsal pad, surgery
I. Hallux Valgus: An enlargement of the medial eminence (osseous—cartilage), most commonly occurs at the metatarsophalangeal joint.
Etiology: Shoe with narrow toe box, pes planus, metatarsus primus varus, joint laxity
Clinical: Painful lateral deviation of the great toe at metatarsal joint
Management: Proper shoe wear, surgery
J. Jones' Fracture: Fracture of the base of the 5th metatarsal of the foot
Clinical: Pain, tenderness and swelling over the lateral border of the foot
• Swelling and erythema is also common
Management: Short-leg cast

(continued)

TABLE 8–4: Common Conditions and Management (Continued)
K. Köhler's Disease: An osteonecrosis of the tarsal navicular bone, common in young age
Clinical: Medial midfoot pain, pain exacerbated with activity and relieved with rest
Management: Rest, analgesics PRN, casting, surgery
L. Osteochondritis Dissecans: An osteochondral fracture from talar dome that affects the articular surface of the talus, which articulates with the tibia
Clinical: Ankle pain with intermittent swelling and grinding s/p trauma or avascular necrosis
• **Classification:**
Stage 1—Subchondral compression
Stage 2—Incomplete osteochondral fracture
Stage 3—Compete nondisplaced osteochondral fracture
Stage 4—Displaced fragment
Management: Rest, activity restriction, reduce weight wearing, casting, surgical repair
M. Plantar Fasciitis
Etiology: Chronic inflammation of the plantar fasciitis, microadhesions
Clinical: Heel pain worse with first step and improves with ambulation
• Tenderness noted over calcaneus exacerbated with dorsiflexion of the toe
Management: Anti-inflammatory medication, splint, stretching, proper orthotics, steroid + lidocaine injection, surgery

(continued)

TABLE 8–4: Common Conditions and Management (Continued)

N. Retrocalcaneal Bursitis: Pain over posterior calcaneus

Management: Anti-inflammatory medication and proper orthotics with padding over posterior hill

O. Tarsal Tunnel Syndrome: Entrapment of the posterior tibial nerve. Pain radiating to sole and toes

Etiology: Tendon sheath ganglion, tarsal tunnel lipoma, exostosis impinging on the nerve, neurilemoma within tarsal tunnel

Management: Treat underlying lesion, anti-inflammatory medication, splint, proper orthotics

TABLE 8–5: Special Tests

A. Anterior Drawer Test

Indications

• Lateral ankle sprain evaluation

Advantages in evaluation of ankle stability

• Most sensitive test, least painful test

Technique

• Foot in slight plantar flexion

• Brace anterior shin with left hand

• Pull heel anteriorly with right hand

• Positive test findings

  • Laxity and poor endpoint on forward translation

Anterior drawer sign

Testing for integrity of anterior talofibular ligament

Fibula
Tibia
Talus
Anterior talofibular ligament

Calcaneofibular ligament
Calcaneus

(continued)

TABLE 8–5: Special Tests (Continued)

B. External Rotation Test

Indications

- Suspected syndesmotic sprain of the ankle

Technique

- Patients knee flexed over edge of table
- Examiner stabilizes leg proximal to ankle
- Examiner uses other hand to grasp plantar foot
- Rotate foot externally relative to tibia

Interpretation

- Pain on external rotation suggests syndesmotic sprain

C. Inversion Test

Indications

- Check stability of lateral ligament complex
  (anterior talofibular & calcaneofibular ligament)

Technique

- Examiner cups heel of affected foot in one hand while the opposite hand stabilizes the anterior part of distal tibia and fibula
- To check for anterior talofibular ligament, examiner maximally plantarflexes the ankle and then inverts the rearfoot
- To check for calcaneofibular ligament, examiner maximally dorsiflexes the ankle and then inverts the rearfoot

Interpretation

- Abnormal when 10–15 degrees more inversion than opposite side

(continued)

TABLE 8–5: Special Tests (Continued)

Inversion test

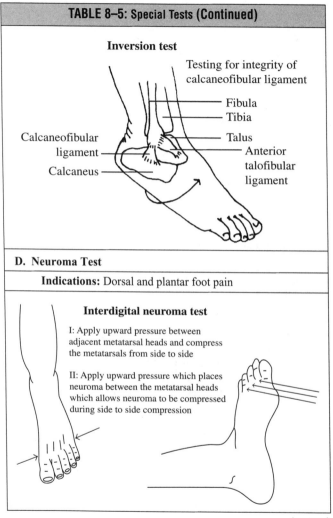

Testing for integrity of
calcaneofibular ligament

Fibula
Tibia

Calcaneofibular
ligament

Talus
Anterior
talofibular
ligament

Calcaneus

D. Neuroma Test

Indications: Dorsal and plantar foot pain

Interdigital neuroma test

I: Apply upward pressure between
adjacent metatarsal heads and compress
the metatarsals from side to side

II: Apply upward pressure which places
neuroma between the metatarsal heads
which allows neuroma to be compressed
during side to side compression

(continued)

TABLE 8–5: Special Tests (Continued)

E. Ottawa Ankle Rule

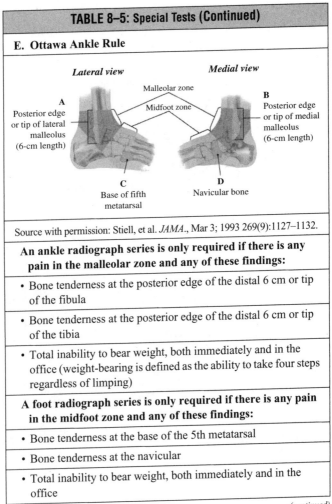

Lateral view　　　　　*Medial view*

Malleolar zone

A
Posterior edge
or tip of lateral
malleolus
(6-cm length)

Midfoot zone

B
Posterior edge
or tip of medial
malleolus
(6-cm length)

C
Base of fifth
metatarsal

D
Navicular bone

Source with permission: Stiell, et al. *JAMA.*, Mar 3; 1993 269(9):1127–1132.

An ankle radiograph series is only required if there is any pain in the malleolar zone and any of these findings:

- Bone tenderness at the posterior edge of the distal 6 cm or tip of the fibula

- Bone tenderness at the posterior edge of the distal 6 cm or tip of the tibia

- Total inability to bear weight, both immediately and in the office (weight-bearing is defined as the ability to take four steps regardless of limping)

A foot radiograph series is only required if there is any pain in the midfoot zone and any of these findings:

- Bone tenderness at the base of the 5th metatarsal

- Bone tenderness at the navicular

- Total inability to bear weight, both immediately and in the office

(continued)

TABLE 8–5: Special Tests (Continued)

F. Talar Tilt

Technique

- Brace heel with left hand
- Invert foot with right hand
- Compare to opposite side

Signs of ankle joint instability

- Joint laxity
- Lack of endpoint on translation

Talar tilt

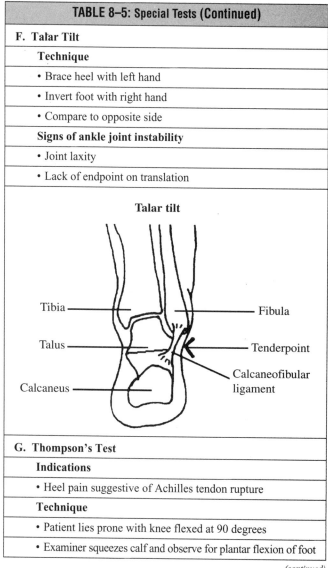

Tibia — Fibula

Talus — Tenderpoint

Calcaneofibular ligament

Calcaneus —

G. Thompson's Test

Indications

- Heel pain suggestive of Achilles tendon rupture

Technique

- Patient lies prone with knee flexed at 90 degrees
- Examiner squeezes calf and observe for plantar flexion of foot

(continued)

TABLE 8–5: Special Tests (Continued)

Interpretation

- Normal response: Plantar flexion as reflex response
- Achilles tendon rupture: Plantar flexion absent

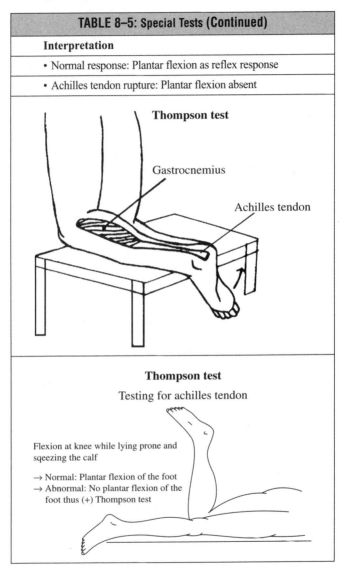

Thompson test

Gastrocnemius

Achilles tendon

Thompson test

Testing for achilles tendon

Flexion at knee while lying prone and sqeezing the calf

→ Normal: Plantar flexion of the foot
→ Abnormal: No plantar flexion of the foot thus (+) Thompson test

9
Spine

FIGURE 9–1: Anatomy

A Spine musculature

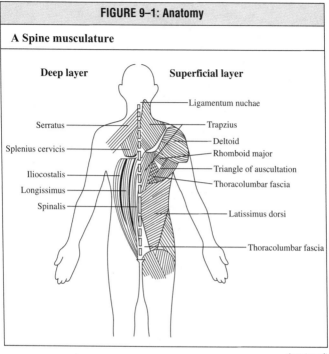

Deep layer

Superficial layer

- Ligamentum nuchae
- Serratus
- Trapzius
- Splenius cervicis
- Deltoid
- Rhomboid major
- Iliocostalis
- Triangle of auscultation
- Longissimus
- Thoracolumbar fascia
- Spinalis
- Latissimus dorsi
- Thoracolumbar fascia

(continued)

FIGURE 9–1: Anatomy (Continued)

Spine musculature

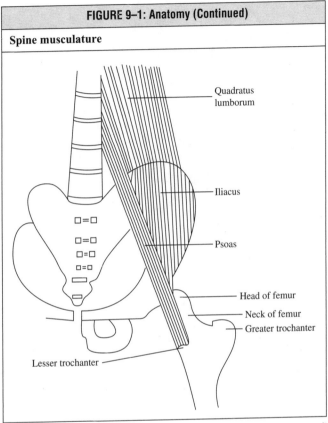

(continued)

FIGURE 9–1: Anatomy (Continued)

Spine pathology

Back muscle and nerve roots

Anterior   *Posterior*

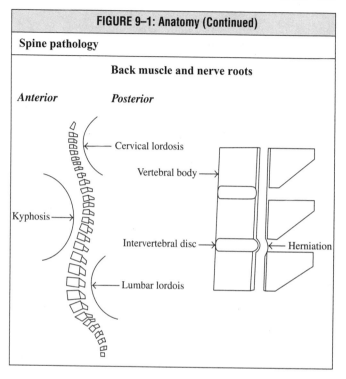

TABLE 9–1: Assessment of Injury

• **Detailed history (including occupational and psychological stressors) red flags**
• Bowel or bladder dysfunction or weakness
• Neurological dysfunction
• History of malignancy
• Cauda equina syndrome
• Age >50 yrs
• Fever
• Unintentional weight loss
A. Inspection: Swelling, erythema, discoloration, deformity, laceration
B. Palpation: Bones and soft tissue—tenderness, deformity, effusion, trigger points
C. Range of motion: Passive and active
D. Motor
E. Sensory (see Chapter 1)
F. Deep tendon reflex (see Chapter 1)
I. Straight leg raise test
II. Gait, heel-toe walk, and squat and rise
III. Stance
IV. Waddell sign

TABLE 9–2: Diagnostic Approaches
Imaging Studies:
• Radiograph: AP, lateral (Swimmer's view for C7–T5)
• MRI
• CT scan
• DEXA scan
• Myelography
• Bone scan
Lab Studies:
• CBC with diff
• ESR, CRP
• Blood C&S
• PSA
• HLA–B27
Other Studies:
• EMG
• NCS
• TB skin test
AP—Antero-posterior; CBC—Complete blood count; CRP—C-Reactive protein; EMG—Electromyogram; ESR—Erythrocyte sedimentation rate; NCS— Nerve conduction study

TABLE 9–3: Common Conditions and Management

A. Ankylosing Spondylitis

- Common in ages between 15 and 40 yrs. It may present with morning stiffness with decreased range of motion of back and/or tenderness over SI joint.

- May be associated with elevated ESR, positive HLA–B27.

- X-ray may show bamboo spine

B. Back Strain

- Common in ages between 20 and 40 yrs.

- Presents with lower back/buttock/posterior thigh pain. Pain usually increased with activity. Localized tenderness and limited spinal motion.

C. Cauda Equina Syndrome: It is a collection of intradural L2–L4 nerve roots.

- Presents as an urinary retention, bladder and bowel incontinence, saddle anesthesia, severe and/or progressive weakness of lower extremities.

D. Compression Fracture

- The pain associated with compression fractures varies in quality from dull, aching to sharp pain. It is aggravated with sitting and activity. During sleep, muscle spasm may occur. The pain from the acute phase of compression fractures usually lasts 4–6 weeks. If the pain is present for a longer time, another cause should be investigated.

- The majority of compression fractures of the vertebra are discovered incidentally on abdominal or chest x-rays. Two-thirds of fractures are usually asymptomatic. It can lead to height loss, which in turn leads to kyphosis.

- Most women who are symptomatic can not relate a history of preceding injury or trauma. These patients typically present with history of lifting, bending, or coughing prior to experiencing back pain.

(continued)

TABLE 9–3: Common Conditions and Management (Continued)

E. Disk Herniation (See Figure 9–1 C)

- Herniated disc occurs when there is a weakening of the ligamentous fibers caused by the degeneration and intervertebral pressure of the fibers. This in turn creates a tear in the annulus leading to a prolapse of the nucleus pulposus. If a nerve root is pressed on by the herniated nucleus pulposus then radicular symptoms ensue.

- Pain presents as sharp, burning, or shooting paresthesia in leg. Pain increased with bending or sitting and decreased with standing.

F. Episacroiliac Nodules AKA "Back Mice"

- Episacroiliac nodules are mobile fibrofatty nodules located in the presacral region. They can be an occasional cause of low back pain. Local anesthetic with or without steroids can be injected into the nodules and may be beneficial in those with persistent pain. Surgery is rarely indicated to remove these nodules.

G. Malignancy

- Throbbing, slowly progressive localized pain and tenderness with or without neurologic abnormalities and or fever. Pain may increase with cough or recumbency.

- Most common malignancy that metastasize to spine are multiple myeloma, breast, lung, thyroid, kidney, and prostate.

- May have abnormal serum electrophoresis, urinary Bence-Jones protein.

H. Osteoarthritis

- Osteoarthritis of the spine does not commonly cause back pain. However, osteoarthritis leads to degeneration of the spine predisposing patients to spinal stenosis which is a common cause of back pain in elderly.

(continued)

TABLE 9–3: Common Conditions and Management (Continued)
• If a patient has low back pain and history of osteoarthritis always test the range of motion of the hip; because osteoarthritis of the hip can present with low back pain.
• X-rays should not only include the spine also an AP view of the pelvis.

I. Piriformis Syndrome

• This occurs when the sciatic nerve is compressed by the piriformis muscle due to contracture or spasm. Physical symptoms include buttock tenderness or pain and are usually exacerbated with sitting for a prolonged period of time.
• Findings on physical examination are as follows:
Sciatic notch tenderness
Buttock pain with hip abduction against resistance
Pain with hip flexion
Pain with hip internal rotation

J. Spinal Infection

• Localized tenderness with fever and may display neurological abnormalities. Usually associated with decreased spine motion

K. Spinal Stenosis

• Spinal stenosis is also known as neurogenic claudication occurs most commonly in the elderly. It is caused most commonly by arthritis that leads to disc degeneration. There is narrowing of one or more areas in the spine and this can lead to pressure on the nerves that branch out from that area causing radicular symptoms.
• Pain may present as shooting pain or pins and needles sensation. Pain usually increased with walking, especially uphill. Pain decreased with sitting.

(continued)

TABLE 9–3: Common Conditions and Management (Continued)

L. Spondylolisthesis

- Spondylolisthesis is the anterior slippage of one vertebra on another. It can be inherited or acquired. Most commonly it occurs from recurrent stress on the pars interarticularis (posterior elements of the spine). It commonly involves L5 on S1 or L4 on L5.

- Pain usually presents as back or posterior thigh. Pain increased with activity or bending.

M. Spondylolysis

- Spondylolysis is a defect/stress fracture of pars interarticularis of the vertebrae. This most commonly occurs at L5 and believed to be caused by repeated microtrauma and also may be inherited.
- Spondylolysis typically occurs from repeated microtrauma especially with repeated or excessive hyperextension of the lumbar spine. This is seen most commonly in adolescent athletes such as divers, soccer players, gymnasts, weight lifters, dancers, and football players. Also, it may be present at birth whereby there were malformations of the facet joints. Positive family history predisposes an individual to spondylolysis in addition to S1 spina bifida. There are some patients who have no identifiable risk factors.

N. Others

- **Abdominal aortic aneurysm (AAA):** May present with back pain not alleviated with rest, pulsatile mass in abdomen and inability to find comfortable position.

- **Gout**

- **Pyelonephritis**

- **Endometriosis**

- **Pancreatitis**

- **Aortic aneurysm**

- **Pelvic inflammatory disease**

TABLE 9–4: Special Tests

Nerve Root and its Action

Nerve root	Action	Motor exam
L3	Squat down and rise up	Hip extension (quadriceps)
L4	Walk on heels	Ankle dorsiflexion
L5	Walk on heels	Great toe dorsiflexion
S1	Walk/stand on toes	Ankle plantar flexion

B. Straight Leg Raise:

Indication: Testing for ipsilateral radicular pain secondary to nerve root compression

Technique: Raise leg with knee extension and dorsiflex the foot (positive test: symptoms occur at >30 degrees)

30 degrees   Straight leg raise

C. Waddell's Signs for Nonorganic Etiology of the Back Pain

Tests	Inappropriate response to test
Palpation	Excessive tenderness to light touch
Axial loading	Light pressure on skull while standing produces back pain

(continued)

TABLE 9–4: Special Tests (Continued)	
Rotation	Rotation of shoulders and pelvis in same plane causes back pain
Distraction	Inconsistent findings when patient is distracted.
Motor	Generalized giving-way weakness ("Cogwheel") on muscle testing
Sensory	Nondermatomal sensory loss
Overreaction	Disproportionate pain response, facial expression or verbalization during examination

Index